Born
UNDER THE
Gaslight

Born UNDER THE Gaslight

A Memoir of My Descent into Borderline Personality Disorder

Cindy Collins

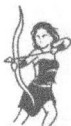

Indomitable Publishing LLC

Indomitable Publishing, LLC
© Cindy Collins, 2019

First Edition

Edited by: The insightful Ellen Miller and Brooks Becker
Cover and text design by: The amazing Lorna Reid
Foreword by: The brilliant Sheila S. Cohen, PhD

Disclaimer: This is a memoir. No events or names have been fabricated. The story and dialog have been recreated as accurately as possible from the author's memory. Although others may recollect said events differently, this is not their story. This is the author's version of events that occurred.

Table of Contents

Forward

✷

This book is about putting words to feelings and experiences. Ms. Collins has demonstrated the importance of having a voice. Her voice is, unfortunately, the voice of many children and adults living with and/or suffering from childhood trauma. I applaud the author for her bravery in her writing and in sharing her life story with others; so that others do not feel so alone. She shines a light on intense and often taboo topics; child sexual abuse and emotional abuse of children by parents. Her writing is poignant and laced with humor as she recounts her journey from childhood to adulthood through the lens of abuse. Her bravery and vulnerability validate for survivors their feelings of shame, guilt, confusion or 'craziness', the difficulty in subsequent adult relationships and the eternal desire to be loved by an abusing parent. Ms. Collins further touches on system deficits that make the road to recovery challenging including barriers to obtaining therapy and to finding counselors that understand trauma. Cindy Collins is a single candle who, in her book, has allowed us to see what goes on in the dark space behind the house window where a child lived, grew up, dreamt and suffered.

∽

This book is about gaslighting. Gaslighting is lying. Gaslighting is lying with the intent of or for the purpose of emotional manipulation. Gaslighting is traumatic for the collective psyche. It is especially traumatic when it is carried out by a parent(s) towards a child(children). Early trauma (whether physical, sexual or emotional) has long-lasting effects on a person's psychological development and health. When gaslighting and trauma happen between a caregiver and a child it has a significant and detrimental impact. A secure attachment between a child and a caregiver provides a base from which that child learns about relationships, love, themselves, and explores the world. It is the foundation for psychologically healthy development. A secure attachment also involves emotional and reciprocal attunement between a child and a caregiver. That is, being in sync with each other and having one's physical and emotional needs understood and met. Bowlby and others have written much about the importance of attachments and attunement. When attachments are not secure, children develop in maladaptive ways, in part because of their attempts to cope. Gaslighting interferes with safe and secure attachments and can contribute to children falling victim to further abuse.

∽

This book is about abuse suffered by many children. We now know that trauma alters the structure of the brain and the stress hormones do not function in a typical manner. For example, one speech center of the brain, Broca's area, is decreased in size making it particularly harder to put feelings and thoughts into words. The amygdala which is the emotional area that warns of danger gets out of equilibrium with the thinking part of the brain; ensuring that emotions will be overwhelming, intense and hard to control. Further, stress hormones (like adrenaline) take a long time to return to a normal level or be in balance again. The heightened level of hormones contributes to a trauma survivor often feeling on alert. This influences the fight/flight response that is normal in the face of trauma or disaster. For traumatized persons there is a loss of balance of these things resulting in easily reliving the trauma. In fact, the physiological effects of trauma last long after the trauma has passed. If the trauma is ongoing, the impact is especially detrimental on healthy development. Clearly, trauma makes internal changes and thus changes the way one approaches the external world. Dr. Bessel Van der Kolk, in his book <u>The Body Keeps the Score</u>, explains these changes that result from trauma.

∽

This book is about highlighting the importance of understanding and talking about child sexual abuse and child trauma. The Center for Disease Control (CDC) statistics show that about one in four girls and one in 13 boys experience sexual abuse at some point in childhood. Further, 90% of child sexual abuse is perpetrated by someone the child or child's family knows. A recent CDC study assessing adults found that 60% of those surveyed had experienced at least one traumatic event during childhood. The study was conducted from 2015 through 2017 and involved over 140,000 adults across 25 states. Much research, including this one, details the long-lasting impact of even one traumatic event on putting victims at a higher risk of chronic health problems as well as emotional and psychological difficulties. Childhood abuse and trauma is a national epidemic that deserves to be recognized, talked about and prioritized. Ms. Collins has done this in an honest, poignant and understandable way.

∽

Finally, this book is about resilience. Not only does Ms. Collins show her own resilience but the book leaves us with the hope of resilience within children and all survivors. Every life is a puzzle with many pieces and putting those pieces together to make us whole takes a lifetime of understanding. The puzzle starts when we are little with attachments to caregivers and as we grow and change and build our internal world, we realize our own powers. Ms. Collins in this book shines the light on childhood resilience and the internal power of the human soul.

∽

As a child psychologist with over twenty years of work with children and teens and young adults, many of whom have experienced abuse and traumatic events, I believe this book is very powerful. It is a must read for survivors of abuse and for all of us working with people who have experienced trauma.

Thank-you Ms. Cindy Collins for sharing your story with us so that we may learn, understand, heal and find the light in ourselves and others.

Sheila S. Cohen, Ph.D.
Clinical Psychologist

Acknowledgments

☀

Early on, I learned that my whole life revolved around this mysterious entity of The Neighbors. I never knew The Neighbors. What I did know was they were factored into the equation of life. It was the constant statements from my mother reinforcing these ideals. "What will the neighbors think?" "Change your clothes before the neighbors see you." "Keep your voice down, or the neighbors will hear you screaming."

I never knew The Neighbors, but, more important, they never knew my family. They never knew what was happening on their street. Right next door was a house of horror, and they indeed never knew. This book could have been dedicated to those that supported me during my life. But instead, it's dedicated to The Neighbors. This is the story that was carefully concealed from you. This is the story that can happen even if you do grow up with neighbors watching. This is for The Neighbors.

Introduction

✻

Billy made sure to take the license plate off my car before getting in. He knew we were about to play my favorite game. My LED bouncing star headband lit up my car with flashing lights begging to attract attention. We would speed around town luring the police to chase us. They were the most fun to race. They wouldn't drive down one-way streets the wrong way or blatantly fly through stop signs. We would, which is why we never lost. This was how we practiced for street racing. The LSD would amplify my senses, giving me tunnel vision. Pumped up on speed, shifting gears so fast that I could jump gears, I could breathe. I drove the way my brain operated... fast, reckless, and out of control. This was the mind of a borderline, and it was just a random Tuesday.

I was diagnosed with Borderline Personality Disorder in my twenties. I never understood the extent to which it ran my life or the degree of dysfunction that it entailed. Only in my forties did I start to work on getting help managing it. By that time, I learned I was also diagnosed with Dissociative Amnesia Disorder and Post Traumatic Stress Disorder, including side effects of depression and anxiety. I was pretty much one face slap away from completely transcending into Dissociative Identity Disorder. Often, I think how sad it is that I never completed that transformation. Maybe then I would have had more friends growing up, even if only in my head.

When I heard the term Borderline, I always thought it meant on the border of sanity and insanity. I felt like I was one thread away from becoming completely unhinged. In reality, it is a condition where you have no coping skills or emotion regulation. So, if you feel anger or sadness, you feel it on the tsunami scale. Suicide and the longing for death are the natural partners to your internal level of sadness. "Almost 80% of those with BPD report a history of suicide attempts, and suicide deaths range between 8–10%. This rate is fifty times greater than that found in the general population, according to a 2014 analysis of BPD research by the Substance Abuse and Mental Health Services Administration (SAMHSA)." (Sack, D., 2015). Having no control of your emotions, while constantly feeling out of control, would make anyone want to take a break from the living.

People with Borderline Personality Disorder have

no sense of self. Your identity becomes reliant on those around you. Being identity-dependent on others causes your world to collapse in their absence. They become your mirror to let you know who you are. You become the ultimate chameleon blending with groups just trying to fit in. The thinking style is extreme in only seeing things as black or white. Grey does not exist.

My extreme fits of rage and anger made it easy for my family to dismiss me as the "crazy one." Funny thing about the so-called crazy ones is that sometimes, it's people that made us that way. Trauma is the only factor that could have created all these mental illnesses that I had to learn to deal with. Trauma is what I had in spades. To me, the word "trauma" is synonymous with the word "family." And my mother was indeed the head of that family.

Science has discovered that children's brains are neurologically altered by trauma. *American Nurse Today* states, "Women who were sexually abused as children show significantly diminished brain volume on brain scans. The structure and function of the hippocampus (responsible for learning and memory), for example, are different when compared to individuals who weren't traumatized. The medial prefrontal cortex, amygdala, and other neural circuitry of the brain are also changed" (Severson, 2012).

That indeed is a drop in the bucket of the damage done when a child is impacted with trauma during formative years. I wonder what my brain would have ended up like growing up in a different house. I endured so many types of abuse that it would be difficult to pinpoint which occurrence fried my neuropathways' trip to wellness. What I do know is my rage, my anger is always directed at my mother.

The Creation of a Borderline

✸

Lonely. Lonely is how I would describe my childhood. My parents would take motorcycle trips across the United States of America and leave my brother and me home alone for weeks at a time. They would instruct the movie-rental place to give us whatever we liked. They would settle the bill when they returned. Blank checks were left on the counter in case any emergency occurred such as furnace or water heater problems. Sometimes bills were left on the counter for us to mail out for them in their absence. I was enrolled in elementary school at the time. My brother was seven years older than me but still not a responsible adult. It's hard to be sure what age I was when certain things happened. Trauma victims frequently have difficulties determining ages. It's like our brains want to block out the fact that horrific things can happen to a young child.

Family vacations occurred very infrequently. The result was the same whether we traveled to Florida or Tennessee. I would end up sitting in a hotel room by myself watching TV. My parents would leave me a pile of quarters for the vibrating hotel bed as my entertainment. They would stay out late walking the strip. Instructions were issued to stay in the hotel room and not answer the door to anyone. After they left, my brother would go out to meet up with townie kids. I preferred it when he left. Most nights he would spend masturbating and tasting his own sperm. He was never a balanced individual. This was the fun-filled vacation time to make up for the daily terror that we endured at home.

Abandonment is a contributing factor in creating Borderline Personality Disorder. From the beginning there was basic neglect and child negligence. Looking back, it's easy to see how leaving a child alone in hotel rooms was so dangerous. There was an outdoor river that ran right next to our hotel. They never worried about their unsupervised kids drowning from playing in the river. They never worried about someone stealing their children. To worry about someone implies that you care about that person. Being a clumsy child, I would accidentally fall and break my wrists four separate times. One of these bone breaks did occur on vacation.

Sexual abuse is another component in creating

Borderline Personality Disorder. Science has established that childhood molestation alters the brain, affecting your functioning into adulthood. Childhood abuse causes developmental delays such as survivors of abuse incurring more medical expenses from related health-care issues. They are more likely to abuse drugs and alcohol and have an eating disorder or other suicidal or destructive behavior (Butler, 2016). My sexual abuse, combined with childhood neglect, were contributing factors to the development of my Borderline Personality Disorder.

It's easy to discuss the facts that created a borderline. The truth remains that there were people behind those damaging actions. Was it one person that created a borderline? Was it multiple people that created a borderline? Let's start down the road and see who played the role of the borderline creator.

∞

Before being saddled with children on vacation, my parents would have our grandparents watch over us. My mother always liked my dad's parents better than her own. Maybe it was easier to pretend to be a decent person around strangers. My dad's mother, Joy, and father, Paul, always had bluegrass music playing, which was annoying to me. To this day, I still cannot listen to bluegrass. No real loss in my mind.

Being left with Paul and Joy always came with a set of rules. My mother always gave me a weird list to follow before she left. She always instructed me to not "run around in my cotton Strawberry Shortcake nightgown." She instructed Tim to watch over me and not leave me unattended. Before any abuse or traumatic events occurred, my mother had her doubts but regardless, she rolled the dice. She gambled with my safety for her ability to take a road trip vacation to the Grand Canyon. No healthy-minded adult would have an issue with a child in a nightgown. Of course, most adults wouldn't trade their child's safety to go on vacation.

While staying with the grandparents, I had a rash on my leg. Mother specifically told me that only Joy could apply the medicinal cream. I was never to allow Paul to apply the cream to my lower leg. As an adult, I would later find medical records showing that the rash was shingles. Shingles is common in senior citizens but rare in children. Children with low immune systems from high-stress environments are more prone to shingles.

No spoiler here to learn that Paul was a child molester. He had molested his own daughter prior to me. The family had known this, and it was overlooked as they were dubbed "our babysitters." He pulled me up to sit on his lap and placed me on his other hand. I was restrained when I tried to leave. His fingers rubbed at my pants, pushing on my pubic area, causing me pain. While grabbing my chest, he asked me if I liked it. Finally, when he let me free, I went to do what every after school special tells you to do. I told an adult. I had seen the specials. I knew he did a "bad touch," and I was instructed to tell. What the specials don't tell you is what to do if the adult tells you to keep your mouth shut. Joy told me to keep my mouth shut.

Joy made sure to instruct my brother to keep his mouth quiet since he was there when I told Joy. She told me to push it out of my mind and forget it. Then, as a bonus, Paul pulled me aside to yell at me for telling. He told me how he could get thrown out of the house or divorced, and it would be all my fault. I cried. He grabbed my arms, shaking me all while blaming me for everything. First, Joy told me that if I told my parents it would be my fault my brother and I could no longer visit. Then Paul blamed me for causing marital problems. The term victim-blaming gets darker and more vile when applied to shaming a child.

I confided in the only friend I had at the time. It was a neighborhood girl that I rode three-wheel tricycles with. She stated that he had also painfully grabbed her, pulling her on his lap. She no longer wanted to go with me to my grandparents' house. I lost the first friend I had known. I wrote all about this event in my diary, which my lovely mother would read later.

One would think that a child would be rescued when the diary was read. It was precisely the opposite. No cops were called, and no police report was filed. I believe this was when my value as a human was set on a descending path. My mother made the situation all about her and my father. She stated that supposedly, Paul had made a pass at her. No one would ever have a struggle without my mother having one to match. She also stated how the family had to support my father as he tried to rebuild his relationship with Paul after this "break in trust." I was now branded as the "difficult child" because I did not want to visit the grandparents. I was called selfish because I wasn't supportive of my father and his struggles. I was called the cold, unfeeling child because I didn't recognize mother's struggle of rebuilding the family. This family break was now all the fault of a child.

The compromise my mother came up with was to leave me in the car while they visited Paul and Joy inside the house. Having a child in the vehicle did not prevent them from spending hours inside Paul and Joy's house. On the hot summer days, the leather car seats were fire on my legs. My mother would leave a window cracked, but it offered little relief. Living on air from cracked windows, I had become the equivalent of the family dog.

At the end of every visit, Paul would make it a point to come outside, waving goodbye while laughing at me. Sometimes he would come out and tap on the window and laugh. Other times he would come out and bang on the window demanding that I get out of the car. Sometimes my parents and brother would watch the car interactions from the porch; other times they would not. Terror from the tapping glass sound shook through my body. A single pane of glass seemed so fragile in my mind. I felt trapped and vulnerable every visit. The constant on-edge feeling, the looking over my shoulder, the inability to get comfortable, that would last forever. The cracked windows, combined with the laughing and verbal torment, would add to my psychological break. I always choose to stay locked in the car with the window cracked. Time after time, I was viewed as an animal behind glass, their own personal zoo animal.

My mother's other concern was the neighbor girl I played with. They knew Paul had also molested her. My parents feared she would tell her parents and create a lawsuit. At no time was empathy or horror at the abuse of children a concern. It was all about how they would be perceived by others. My only friend was taken from me. I was instructed that I was no longer allowed to play with her. Just like that, I fell back into the void of loneliness.

My alienation from others was further expanded on by my mother. She had told her side of the family about Paul molesting me. They were instructed to not touch me or hug me for fear of misinterpretation. Everyone was suddenly scared of being accused of child molestation from a goodbye hug. Kids with lice received more affection from family than I did. Blaming and punishing the child for the actions of an adult is reprehensible. I'm sure that's what created my social awkwardness as a child. I now lacked socialization skills I was supposed to learn in my formative years. I was becoming developmentally delayed. All I had learned was isolation.

The grandparents on both sides were no longer options as babysitters to watch us when our parents traveled. My parents loved to travel, preferably without their children. They had a neighbor friend watch us for a bit. That stopped the moment she scolded my parents, saying they shouldn't be traveling so much with small children at home. That friendship ended, as with anyone that came out on the children's side. That left my brother as the sole babysitter option.

My brother was always awkward. Super skinny with glasses and mousey features, he was never the cool kid. He bought into the difficult child brand my parents had placed on me. I believe his hatred of me grew deeper with every trip my parents took. He was regularly annoyed by the family dynamic revolving around me. No brotherly love would develop by tasking him with the job of raising a child. He had to cook for us and run the house, and he wasn't even in high school. I got used to eating a lot of mac n cheese since he knew very few recipes.

My parents had made me his burden. This fueled his resentment toward me and further solidified my isolation. He viewed me as the damaged, abused sister. Maybe this made it easier for him to disregard me as a human. I was still a human that wanted the most basic need of human interaction. Instead of interacting with me on a healthy level, my brother opted to teach me that my body was a tool to barter with. It was a separate object, a commodity. If I wanted a playmate, then I had to make it worth his while.

I wanted so much for my brother to play Strawberry Shortcake dolls with me. Those dolls were my favorite. I even had the special Strawberry Shortcake cake mix for my Easy-Bake Oven. I would make cakes from water and a light bulb to go along with our mac n cheese. But to get him to play dolls, I had to agree to let him place a plastic baggie inside my vagina filled with whipped cream and eaten out. I did not understand why anyone would want to do that. The internal coldness felt unbearable. Here was another family member that was hurting me. The pain was in a place that should have been protected by those that are supposed to love you most.

He would ignore my cries of pain while yelling at me to stop struggling. He attempted to convince me that it's just like the Operation board game. He said that by playing his game first, then he would play my choice next. Again, I was pushed to not be the difficult child. I was to be used for someone else's perversions. According to him, I owed him. Everyone's struggles always seemed more important than my own. He was now the one in charge, and I had no choice. I could not even have a safe home environment. As I lay back, another piece of my childhood sanity drifted away. I was deemed worthless by those who were supposed to value me above all others.

I was not even eight years old, and I was already feeling suicidal. I felt an immense feeling of shame and guilt from my life and was unable to comprehend these emotions or their origins. I was too young. I just knew my brain felt unhinged, and I no longer wanted to live. This feeling would permanently follow me into adulthood. Kids this age are disappointed with missing the ice cream truck. I was dealing with the disappointment of being alive in this life. Contemplating life and death is a complex subject on its own. Now imagine processing it with the mind of a child who has damaged neurological development as a result of childhood abuse.

My brother would try to encourage me to make friends to invite them over to our parent free house. His appetite for sexual perversion was widening from me to outsiders. I was to look the other way while he molested others. In exchange, they could stay and play dolls with me. The house was now being run as a human trafficking sex location, and I was the bait to lure girls in.

Needless to say, eventually I gave up on having friends. The girls would beg me to help them, but I was a child with no adult to turn to for help. Their faces still haunt me. All I could do was to stop trying to make friends. Further down in isolation I descended. I wonder if my brother would have learned predatory behavior if the family had spoken out against Paul.

Later the secret of my brother being a predator

would also come out. I confided in my mother, looking for understanding and support. She decided to take a page from Joy and tell me to keep my mouth shut about what had been happening. She even kept that information from my father. She encouraged me to forget about it and pretend it didn't happen.

The constant gaslighting was one of my mom's specialties. Gaslighting is the ultimate form of abuse, in which the perpetrator causes the victim to lose their identity and self-worth while maintaining power over them. Karyl McBride, Ph.D. states, "[Gaslighting] is a form of verbal and psychological abuse that is insidiously cruel, with the intention of making a person doubt their own sanity. It destabilizes you and can make you wonder about your own memory or perception of reality" (McBride 2018). The constant questioning of reality makes one feel like they are indeed the crazy one. The stage was set to ensure that I would obtain Borderline Personality Disorder in this invalidating environment.

How does one describe my mother? I can tell you how the public sees her. She was a band booster parent when I was in high school color guard. She showed up to all my dance recitals. She was a referee when I was on the swim team. An active church member, she raised her kids in church. Her motorcycle group does toy drives and feeds senior citizens at Christmas time. She created a kindness award to be handed out, encouraging kindness to others. She competed in the Mrs. America

Pageant. She portrays the archetype of the faithful, loving wife of one husband for fifty years. Sending constant presents to my brother's kids, she is the doting grandma. The collection of these actions and more caused her to be inducted into her hometown's hall of fame. None of this is what I will remember her for. None of this is as it seems on the surface. I would have preferred the cruelty of Joan Crawford as a mommy dearest figure.

As a child, I used to believe that my mother was the most beautiful woman ever created. She would wear these beautiful floral dresses to church. Her long blonde hair was tied with a matching satin ribbon, creating the perfect accent headband. The delicate girl next door features paired perfectly with her tall, thin frame. Church service consisted of her sitting between my father and me. She said I was unable to be near him since God might call him to the front of the church to save his soul. I was informed that my sitting by him would be distracting. Even then, there was a competition aspect that I didn't understand. Even before I was known as the damaged, molested daughter.

Mother was viewed as the all-American housewife who stayed at home to watch over and cook for her children. She would make me a drink called sun tea. It was in a large glass jar accented with bright yellow flowers. The container was filled with a murky yellow fluid. The drink would cause my nose to immediately gush blood. She would break out her Bible, tilt my head back, and heal me with the power of God. She told me I had allergies to tea—although this didn't seem to stop her from giving me the tea. This was my induction into the world of Munchhausen by Proxy Syndrome. A better explanation is, "Someone who has MSP may purposely take action to make his or her child sick. They knowingly will expose the child to painful or risky medical procedures, even surgeries. They may deliberately create symptoms in a child. They can do this by withholding food, poisoning or suffocating the child, giving the child inappropriate medicines, or withholding prescribed medicines. Creating these situations can put the child at extreme risk" (Staff, 2018). One would think she would have loved using my molestation for attention. However, she only seemed to like attention for things that she created.

The attention she would create followed me into the school system. Navigating social situations as a child can be tricky. You are learning about school friends and cliques. I was still socially delayed, which made it extra difficult. When other kids would go to recess, I would opt to stay inside with the teacher. Most younger kids strive to blend in and be like everyone else. You want to wear all the trendy labels and be considered normal. This was impossible to achieve in my household. My mother was the master of sabotage. School teachers can only protect you so much. By the time I reached junior high school, bullying was a part of my everyday life. I learned to eat my lunch in bathroom stalls and avoid all social interaction. Kids are ruthless at that age to any kid that is viewed as weak or different.

The clothes my mother sent me to school in might as well have been a huge bullseye on my back. They consisted of things such as leather pants with a gun bullet belt, an all-bright-blue spandex onesie, or a sweater that had rabbits' feet hanging on it. My old-lady-style glasses, complete with attached chain, were the perfect accent to the nightmare that was my wardrobe. Nothing about my clothes was appropriate for any person in any situation. Kids would shove me, put gum in my long brown hair, throw paint on my clothes, and use various other bullying tactics. One day I was held down while condoms were shoved into my mouth. The feeling of suffocation squeezed my chest tight with pain and fear of death. Every day I would come home crying. Every day my mother was there waiting with open arms.

Was this how you raised a kid to be strong? It felt like the equivalent of throwing a kid in the water to teach them how to swim. Strength was something preached about in our household. Quitting anything was for the weak. With a broken arm, I was pushed to finish my swim team events. My mother became a referee to ensure I continued. She tied a garbage bag around my cast and pushed me forward. It was my job to portray to others that it was my idea to continue. If I was to give any verbal pushback, I was reminded about how selfish I was. I was expected to be grateful to have such a mother involved in activities. Otherwise, I would be responsible for her embarrassment. It was known that I had to protect her image for our college-age coach, with whom she seemed to enjoy spending all her extra time.

In the swim team offseason, my mother enrolled me in a dance program. But not just any dance program would do. She chose the same program my school bullies attended. Being bullied wasn't limited to school hours. This would carry over into extracurriculars. While on the swim team, I would have two boys try and tear off my swimsuit while I would scream for help. Mother would scold my brother for not intervening in his friends' attempt at violating me. I would call for my brother to help, but he just stood by laughing at my struggle. He had traded me for a date with the boy's sister. Dance class consisted of girls tripping and shoving me while making it look like an accident. I had transitioned from an activity filled with sexual assault to one filled with physical assault.

The bullying from dance class students would lead to my next broken arm. A girl would shove me, causing me to fall and break my arm. For my dance recital costume, Mother made a matching sequin sleeve. The sleeve was to go over yet another broken-arm cast. Later in life, I would finally be able to quit a program. I quit the high school marching band dance squad; however, this would occur when I became homeless at seventeen. My parents would continue traveling with the marching band. They saw nothing wrong with being the only parents there with no child enrolled. Their support was never contingent on me as much as it was others' perception.

The persona portrayed by mother was far from the truth. The public viewed her as a loving parent. Her true nature was displayed most often over food. My mother was never one to believe in expiration dates. We would have frozen meals in the freezer that were over ten years old. There was food in there that had been discontinued. I had to screen the food that was snacked on by other classmates. It was always amazing to go to others' houses and see that they could randomly eat foods without looking at expiration dates. The most basic need for eating was compromised daily. My father always received his dinner later when he got home from work. This ensured that my dinner time with my mother was extra special since it was unsupervised.

One of her special meals caused me to vomit all over the kitchen table. I was not excused to leave the table, even after explaining how it caused me to be nauseous. I was told it was all in my head and to continue eating it. Gaslighting and invalidating my feelings was not going to make that Salisbury steak any more edible. The smell from coagulated gravy chunks atop burnt expired meat, was enough to turn my stomach.

The body knows when to protect itself by expelling rotten food. After emptying my stomach contents all over the family table, my mother immediately made it for me again. She screamed about how she would continue making the meal until I learned to endure the taste and keep the food in my system. Her rage, combined with insults, accusations, and a burst of chilling laughter, was the stuff of horror films. In a manic frenzy, she cooked up another portion of the Salisbury steak dish. She stated that, obviously, I had done that on purpose to agitate her; therefore, I had to clean up the vast quantities of vomit.

I'm not sure of any elementary-school-age child that can vomit on cue, just to ruin someone's day. Apparently, my mother believed that this was indeed a personal attack on her from her own child. By the third time she made the meal, I was able to keep it down. Later in adulthood, I would read the scene in *Mommy Dearest* (Crawford, 1979) involving her steak incident. All I thought was, *Christina Crawford had it easy.*

After the steak incident, I started hiding my blue plastic retainer case in my sock. I would learn to stuff toxic food in it. Later I could flush it down the toilet and hide the fact that I didn't eat dinner. I got used to not eating very much. Mostly I would eat pieces of bread here and there. Combined with fluids, the bread would swell and counter the feeling of hunger. I was adapting to survive the abuse. I was still only a child.

By the time I entered junior high, my family was in full-blown crisis mode. Well, what they viewed as a crisis anyway. My sexual abuse was never viewed as a problem as much as a secret we had to keep. But now we were dealing with my brother planning on going into the military once out of high school. When he applied to the military, a heart condition was discovered. My mom was going to have one of her politician friends pull some strings to get him into the Air Force despite this fact. But for someone that always got what he wanted, patience was not a learned trait. That chance was wasted when he acted out and got arrested.

My brother had developed a new habit. Every time my parents traveled, he went to jail. Later in life, a therapist would tell me, "Kids who steal from their parents are seeking love." My brother must have needed a lot of love. My father had to repurchase his own tools from the pawn shop three times. My parents would leave town, and my brother would proceed to sell off their items. I can't even count how many times my mother bought back his class ring from the pawn shop. My brother started off by breaking into cars. Eventually, he made a rope ladder with metal rungs and started dropping into businesses at night through their ceilings. I would see him working in my father's garage drilling holes in metal bars. This had become such a normal life for me. I would be left home alone while he was out all night cleaning out local businesses. He would come back and dump out duffle bags full of merchandise. My preteen self would be angry because he wouldn't even let me have a Walkman.

One would think that if every time you left for vacation your kid went to jail, you would stop traveling. Or at the very least start taking your kids with you. My parents did not see it this way. My mother's sister would call them and play the police scanner over the phone for them to hear. They were angry that they would have to cut their trip short to come back home. The embarrassment of explaining to their traveling friends that they had to leave was the main concern. They could hear my brother getting chased down by police dogs. He was running through the night, trying to dump merchandise before getting caught. He always got caught. My mother would pull strings to ensure he got placed in a private jail cell. All her police contacts from charity events were coming in handy. In truth, he was a terrible criminal.

My parents did not see that his behavior reflected on their parenting skills. They were never concerned about my brother's future. They were more upset that others knew what was going on. They felt the phone call by the aunt was an attack. They had family that were telling them their kids needed help. All that ever did was get that family member exiled. Every time I tried to ask extended family for help, my mother would cut us off from them. She would create some fake drama as a cover story encouraging my father to disown his sisters or brothers. She thrived on playing the victim. I was viewed as causing trouble, ruining her name, and it just created a more miserable living situation. Our family was mainly just the four of us now. It seemed easier to contain the scandals if the extended family was cut out.

Now we were continually visiting my brother in jail to be supportive. I was always expected to be supportive of those who assaulted me. It never seemed to matter that they brought their troubles on themselves. I was expected to be empathetic and caring toward those that had preyed on the innocent. Sometimes I would try and argue about how I didn't want to go and be a part of this. The days of me sitting in the car were no longer allowed. My voiced objections branded me the "difficult child," followed by slaps to keep me in line. I was known as the "selfish child" that didn't care about others and their pain. I was the child that had a bad attitude, that was always punished for my lack of family support. But they didn't know what difficult was until I entered high school.

I entered high school at the age of fourteen. I could have graduated by the age of sixteen. Mother enrolled me in summer school every summer even though I didn't need it. She stated it was for me to "get ahead," although when I was able to graduate early, she denied me the option. Summer school and school programs were a way of keeping me busy. It was a way of keeping her in a child-free life when she was not on the open road.

When I wasn't in school, I was completing some obsessive cleaning list that she had created. Typical chores involved washing walls in the house. She would have me pull all the clean dishes out of the cabinets, wash them, and put them back. I would be polishing silverware that wasn't silver. Then I would have to remove the polish off the non-silver silverware. I would have to paint the six-foot privacy fence in the back yard. Mother kept a garden filled with planted plastic flowers. I would have to water the pieces of colorful plastic. Standing with a watering can over plastic flowers makes one question their sanity. The number of cleaning chores was always based on the level of mania my mother was feeling that day. The cleaning was to be balanced with never-ending school classes and extracurricular activities. Most would need cocaine or Adderall to keep the schedule that I was given.

My social skills were still severely underdeveloped, as I had very little interaction with people outside my immediate family. Other girls in junior high were becoming sexually aware and interested in boys. I was still playing with dolls and bedwetting during this time. My social development had been stunted. I would learn later in life that this kind of regressed behavior is common in sexually abused children. It did not stop my family from holding these actions against me and blaming me for my shortcomings.

As I entered high school, an odd transition occurred. School bullying stopped. My braces came off, and I switched to contacts and updated my wardrobe. I had been mowing yards that summer for extra income. This enabled me to buy items that were considered more normal for a child to wear. I was also trying to save money to move out. I was fourteen but already planning my escape. Once the bullies ceased to exist, my mother eagerly filled their place. The open arms that had greeted the crying, bullied preteen were now replaced with face slaps for the teenager. My nose now bled from slaps instead of tea. Her anger and rage episodes only got more amplified.

Suddenly everything I bought was considered flawed by my mother. The daily insults were never-ending. If I purchased band T-shirts, it was followed by statements on how they made me look fat, whorish, or flat-chested. If I bought some cute little earrings, then it was commented on as tacky. The CDs I bought were all viewed as artists with no skills. If I could not afford an item that I wanted, my mother would buy it. She did not buy it for me, but rather for her to wear herself. There were comments made with laughter about how sad it must be that I couldn't buy the item. I would watch her walk around in a pair of boots that I longed for. Sometimes she would buy the exact same dress as me, which ensured that I would never wear it. It was as if I was being punished for not wearing items that would subject me to bullying. Every day I was called a whore or accused of becoming a whore. The irony was that I hadn't even kissed a boy. Yet my mother said my future only consisted of me ending up a whore.

My home was now becoming a war zone, and school was to become my sanctuary. For the first time,

I had something I had never had before. I had made friends. Enrolled nonstop in school and extracurriculars, I practically lived at my high school. One day I got on the school bus, and a girl named Laura asked me to sit with her. Laura was two years ahead of me, but decades ahead of me in life skills. She would tell me later that she asked me to sit with her because she had "sensed the darkness" inside of me. I wasn't sure what she had meant by that, but I soon would learn.

Mother loved Laura. On the outside, Laura seemed like a nice young lady. She would drive around with her fluffy little white dog and would actively go to church. Mother had no idea that Laura was romantically involved with the pastor at her church and actively practiced witchcraft. The 90s was a definitive time for the goth culture to thrive, and Laura inducted me into the scene. She knew how to play the nice girl for families, which made it easy for her to spend time with me. Laura would be the one to introduce me to my first transsexual friend, the gay community, and *The Rocky Horror Picture Show* theater group. It was a group where all clothes were black and clove cigarettes were the only option to smoke. She would buy me my first garter belt with thigh highs and introduce me to wearing corsets. This was the first person that would portray sexuality in a positive light.

My new life consisted of me staying at Laura's as much as possible. I would hide my clothes that had become my new uniform for my secret life. This would be the first identity that I would obtain as a borderline. I dove in headfirst and consumed as much of the culture as I could. Fourteen years old, and I was already running around the city after midnight dressed in a black vinyl corset with gold glitter boots. Surrounded by other lost kids, I was already in a safer environment than I ever was at home.

These new kids held my identity. The borderline black and white thinking had me believe that if I wasn't one of them they would leave me. The idea of losing this life was equivalent to my own death. Luckily, the identity that I obtained was perfect for what I had endured. The friends I was making were ones that were dealing with their own issues. They were trying to navigate what it's like to be a teenage homosexual or a teenage transgender. Or even just being a kid that liked to wear all black and listen to The Cure nonstop. They had their own struggles at home. I admired their strength to fight for their freedom to love who they wanted or wear what they wanted. The *Rocky Horror* theater crowd inspired me to find my voice to fight. And just like that, the lid came off.

For so long, I tried to blend into the background in hopes of being overlooked. I wanted to avoid the hitting, the abuse, and the insults. I was exhausted by the gaslighting in which my mother told me that things didn't happen to me or told me to just forget what did occur. I was exhausted by having a mother wake me up in the middle of the night screaming at me for things that never happened. I couldn't even shower without her randomly dumping buckets of ice water over the top of the curtain. I gave up trying to lock the bathroom door. She would use a coat hanger for popping the lock anyway. My torture was her amusement. Nothing she did ever made sense, which made it impossible to brace yourself for it. I would get woken up with cups of water poured on me. Then it was my job to change my bedsheets since she had made them wet. It was nonstop insanity and yet my daily norm.

What with being constantly on edge, sleep deprived, and continually berated, it's incredible that I even functioned. I was still maintaining passing grades. I knew I had to graduate if I wanted to have any chance of supporting myself after I escaped. The fear of staying longer than necessary in that house, combined with years of being pushed not to quit, made for quite the motivational tool. All our family abuse was staying locked behind closed doors. Now they had an off-the-rails burgeoning borderline, fueled by hormones and empowered by peers.

I gave up trying to hide my new-found life. My goth clothes bled into my every day. I tried to ignore the fact my mother again imitated me. She too started buying identical velvet goth dresses. I dyed my hair purple and used a sewing needle to pierce about every orifice that I possibly could. I began cutting into my skin to feel a release of the internal pain. I was angry. Angry at those who were supposed to protect me and instead failed me. I was angry at having my body used and disregarded. I was angry for my pain being viewed as nothing. I had found my voice, and it was prepared to challenge my mother's voice.

My parents were still traveling and leaving my brother in charge. He had decided to place a lock on his bedroom door after I told him to sleep with one eye open. My parents laughed at him for fearing his little sister. The laughing stopped after I stabbed his hand with a knife. He would get angry that I refused to invite any of my friends over. The day he tried to lock me in my room was the day I set the room on fire. I was willing to die in flames if it meant that I could take everyone with me. I escaped my room and ran down the street to the nearest payphone to call a friend for a ride. My mother had unplugged the phone from the outside phone box to prevent me from calling for help within the house. Still, no matter what battle I won for the day, I always ended up going back into the house for another day of war.

Every day was a battle over how I was the family whore. I was accused continuously of having sex with people. One of my school friends had shown me how to use tampons for my menstrual cycle. This further convinced my mother of my sexual promiscuity. Despite my attempts at showing her my high school health book, she believed that only non-virgins could use tampons. She would even gossip about other people's daughters saying they were sleeping around based on their having tampons. There was no reasoning with this level of crazy.

I was at that age where I needed regular medical treatment. Mother had a history of endometriosis and ended up with a hysterectomy from poor genetics. I was doomed to the same fate. Although she informed me that I had endometriosis, she would never take me for medical treatment. The Munchausen by Proxy, once again, would rear its ugly head. Once a month I would spend the week in bed curled up in agonizing pain. She would bring me cups of hot chocolate that only seemed to flush out my insides. I would ask to go to the doctor. I had learned that birth control could reduce my pain and lessen the symptoms of endometriosis. She just accused me of wanting to go on the pill to be promiscuous. In her mind, all my guy friends were either having sex with me or just wanted me for sex.

Once again, my school friends saved me. My friend Justin told me about a place called Planned Parenthood. He and his girlfriend Erica had been going there for birth control. He said that even if I was a minor I could still get treated. He drove me to my first OB/GYN appointment and held my hand in the waiting room. He sat there as I filled out paperwork asking for detailed descriptions of my blood flow and color of my period blood. He would laugh about how much you really can learn about someone. His jokes helped ease my nervousness. My past with sexual assault didn't exactly have me skipping for joy to the table stirrups. Justin never knew how much his support helped me. He had no idea of my history or my home life. He was just being a friend.

A girl's first appointment to an OB/GYN should be with her mother. I was there with a skateboarder guy from my high school art class. Sabotage, not support, was all that my mother was capable of. More than anything, I just wanted to be healthy. And I also didn't want to be in a vulnerable state once a month. It was already bad enough that I had to drink her hot chocolate. All it ever did was give me explosive diarrhea. It was obviously in the same category as her sun tea. But it's hard to fight back when you are flat on your back crippled with pain.

During my new-patient intake appointment, Planned Parenthood informed me that my mother had called their office about my impending visit. She had a nasty habit of listening in on my phone calls. She told the doctors that I couldn't be treated. She said I was highly unstable. She told the doctor that I was a liar, a thief, and a junkie looking to steal all his drugs. I had to speak with the head doctor and convince him that the fourteen-year-old sitting across from him was not the crazy one. I had to prove to him that the responsible, concerned parent was not what she seemed. I was terrified to meet the doctor. This was my first OB/GYN appointment, and Mother was already setting up roadblocks for it.

The doctor finally came in to meet with me. His

visit with me had been delayed based on the number of phone calls that were incoming from my mother. Apparently convincing the doctor that she was crazy wouldn't be that hard after all. She did that all on her own. They informed her that they would be treating me despite her threatening everything from calling the police to lawsuits. Planned Parenthood was used to bomb threats called in from pro-life organizations. They didn't bat an eye at my mother. The doctor handed me my first paper gown and carefully explained the whole process to me before beginning. I think he understood that I might have been more nervous than his normal patients.

I walked out of Planned Parenthood diagnosed with endometriosis, a prescription for birth control in hand. The doctor thought Depo-Provera would be the best option since I would only have to see a nurse quarterly for a syringe injection. It would be easier to hide and didn't come with the added risk of my mother throwing out birth control pills. He informed me that being on birth control would reduce my future risk of infertility by reducing my endometriosis. I was now having to sneak around just to get healthcare.

Justin did what most of my friends had to do. He dropped me off a few blocks away from my house. I tried to avoid subjecting my friends to my mother. She was quick to greet me after my first OB/GYN appointment. Still convinced that some secret boyfriend had taken me there just to encourage more sexual activity, she greeted me with the usual face slaps and insults. The week that followed consisted of an increased amount of her flipping my room. She was constantly turning out drawers, throwing shelf contents on the floor. All of this was, of course, my responsibility to clean up. She was looking for the birth control pills. The doctor at Planned Parenthood reminds me of how not all heroes wear capes. He knew what he was doing by administering a shot rather than handing me pills.

Ask yourself this question: what is more terrifying than a mother that has episodes of manic rage? It's the question that will keep you up at night. The answer is the kind face. The kind face of the mother gives you hope that maybe inside her is a caring, logical being. Inside perhaps is the mother that you have always searched for. The kind face that suddenly emerged cared about my health as a woman. She explained her concerns about Planned Parenthood. The naive teenager listened about how Planned Parenthood was "just a clinic." She painted the picture of how they were not as medically sophisticated as a legitimate doctor's office. And oh, what a lucky day it was for me. She had decided that it was time for me to get a regular OB/GYN doctor through her insurance. The appointment had already been booked, and we were set to leave.

I was so excited at the idea of being able to use my parents' insurance to cover my healthcare and not have to pay out of pocket. However, I was far less excited to be in stirrups once again so quickly. The medical personnel I met with seemed annoyed and didn't even speak directly to me. It was the complete opposite of my experience at Planned Parenthood. Looking back, I have no idea what had been said to them about me. There was no greeting or explanation. Someone entered the room, told me to lie back, administered the pap test, and left the room. I'm not even sure my visit was an actual annual exam. More than likely, it was some random test for sexually transmitted diseases from my nonexistent sex life.

What I also realize is no insurance in the world has a co-pay of a few hundred dollars. My mother served me with a medical bill of over $300. She stated that this was the copay amount that I was responsible for. It was explained that if I wanted to go to adult doctors, then I could have adult bills. I was being punished for getting medical treatment! She took the payment out of the money that I had been saving for moving out when I was eighteen. As an adult, I realized that she never let me use her insurance. This was all an elaborate attempt to deter me from seeking medical treatment. In the end, all it ever did was cement a permanent love of organizations like Planned Parenthood. They were to become my regular doctors throughout my young adult life.

Now the word "whore" was constantly running through my head. Considering it's the one word I heard daily, how could it not? Although I was on birth control, the idea of sex never held any appeal for me. I never wanted to prove my mother right about anything. Therefore, I had zero interest in sex. I asked one of my best guy friends to take my virginity at the age of fourteen. I just wanted to get rid of it at this point and move on. What should have been a memory of a youthful mile marker was instead considered a burden. I decided after that one time to wait for love before I was to become sexually active. Two years later, I met Chuck.

∞

Chuck was unlike anyone I had met before. He didn't hold the dark, jaded attitude of the goth community. He was like the ultimate playmate. His energy level fed right into my mania and opened up the borderline. People with Borderline Personality Disorder are constantly pushing people away to test limits but then pulling them back out of abandonment fear. It's a never-ending roller coaster of confusion that is triggered when entering a relationship. And Chuck had just bought a ticket to this carnival ride.

You never know how love-starved you are until you are in love. If I could have crawled inside Chuck's skin and lived, I would have. My whole life suddenly involved Chuck. Our mutual friends commented on how they couldn't tell where one of us ended and the other began. We shared everything, including clothes. I would put his long black mohawk up into two pigtails while dressing him in my fishnets. I would run around in his multi-green-striped skater shorts. He shaved my long brown hair into a short matching mohawk. Some days we would dress like Droogs from the movie *A Clockwork Orange* for school. Every day for us was Halloween. He would grab my hand and tango with me down the halls to my next class. I felt free to be as crazy as I felt inside my head. Being with Chuck was the biggest natural high that I had ever felt. Complete euphoria.

We would skip class together and hang out in the rafters above the high school auditorium stage. I would bring snacks for our picnic in the rafters. Chuck would light candles to make it romantic. If any student were to look up, they would have seen two people suspended up high having the most interesting school picnic. We would watch others walk below us unaware of the show above them. Early before class, directly after class, all the time possible we were together. I was addicted and dependent on the feeling of love.

As before, where I was utterly immersed in Laura's life with goth culture, I now abandoned all that to consume Chuck. His parents were annoyed that I pretty much lived at his house, but we didn't care. Sometimes they would discover that Chuck had snuck me into the house so I could stay the night with him. They were not fans. Still, they were more supportive of us than my mother. Although my mother was always worried about me having sex, she wanted me to have a boyfriend. She wanted me to have that person to go to school dances with for school pictures. She was looking for that photo op to keep up with other parents. Perception was still everything. I don't think Chuck is what she had in mind for the person in those future pictures.

I knew Chuck was of Korean American heritage, but I never gave it much thought before bringing him home. In my mind, all that meant was dinner at Chuck's house consisted of Korean cooking. I thought the most prominent aspect my parents would hate would be his punk rock hair or baggy skater clothes. His first visit to my home to meet my parents, my mother immediately pulled me into a separate room. She was yelling in hushed tones about how I should have told her he was "foreign." Then she proceeded to get upset, saying she can't talk to someone who doesn't speak English. I explained how Chuck wasn't "foreign," he was American. I also snapped back how he goes to my school, so obviously he can speak English.

Seeing I wasn't going to cave on this topic, she proceeded to cry. Her famous crocodile tears spilled forward only to be ruined by her words. She explained it was just too hard to look at Chuck since she had all her school friends die in the Vietnam War. I countered again, explaining he's Korean not Vietnamese. Told her to try again. Then she started to say she lost friends in the Korean War and continued to cry. I snapped back that during the time frame of the Korean War, she wasn't even born. Miraculously her tears ceased, and she stared at me firmly stating, "I don't like him." That I believed. Going forward, Chuck was known in my house as "the Chink." I didn't even bother to explain that even her racial slur was incorrect. Nothing was going to come between Chuck and me. I knew that this was forever.

Of the four years I was dating Chuck, I would say year one was the only good year. It was to be the only year that Chuck was faithful. I had secretly given him a key to my parents' house. He would come over and wake me up by playing music. Our days would start to the soundtrack of the Violent Femmes or the Sundays. It was more pleasant than being woken up with cold water thrown on you. My parents were either at work or traveling. My brother was usually in jail, so during the summer it was as if Chuck and I lived together.

Chuck spent that year teaching me how to work on my car. My parents had bought me a used car so they wouldn't have to drive me to all my mandatory activities. At first, I was surprised. Then I learned the decision was based on how other parents were buying cars for their children. They always needed to keep up with other families. My parents refused to teach me basic car maintenance. Mother stated that I didn't need to know how to change a tire. She said I just needed to know how to keep a man around. I opted to learn maintenance skills. Chuck taught me oil changes, tire rotations, spark plug changes: everything I asked to learn. He knew what I was up against at home and was willing to help me with life skills.

Having access to a car, I was also able to add an after-school job to my schedule. I was a grocery bagger at a store down the street from Chuck's. Everything that required a choice factored Chuck into things. Some days I couldn't stand to be at work, because it was time away from him. One day I tied toilet paper around the smoke detectors and lit it on fire. I thought this might be a reason they would close the grocery store. The sensors didn't work so I opted to fake sick so I could leave to spend time with Chuck. I was missing class and work just to spend time with him, and it was smothering to him.

The skills Chuck could not help me with were relationship skills. First loves burn a mark on your heart like no other. But this was more than a first love relationship for me. This was the first love of any kind in my life. I was completely starved for it. Chuck could not feed my hunger. Although I wanted all of his time, I kept randomly pushing him away due to having low self-worth. Then seeing him move on, I would pull him back. This is borderline 101. But with each push-pull, he was harder to get back. Every time I spun more out of control. I would have school counselors pull him out of class so we could "talk about our relationship." Ignoring me wasn't an option. If he passed on a counseling meeting, then I would break into his house in the middle of the night. I would watch him sleep and wait for him to wake up so we could "talk about our relationship."

I would buy him a wedding ring proposing marriage and leave it in his locker. I would paint pictures of him in my own blood. Letters of love written in blood is a typical behavior of those with Borderline Personality Disorder. I opted instead for the artistic approach. My art teacher would have the class gather around my art stating how creative it was to use my own blood as a medium. And who says public education isn't filled with caring, observant teachers. All my photographs taken for my graphic arts class were of Chuck. I would sit outside his house in my car and wait for him to come home. Borderline, stalker, they were one and the same.

During our breaks, Chuck would start to date other girls. I would make friends with the girls and get them to dump him. Although I did not have enough self-worth to keep him, I would not allow others to have him. Often, he would tell girls he was done with me then have sex with them.

While they were naked in his bed, he would call me professing his love. Chuck had learned to play head games and become reckless with other people's hearts. One time I even threw him out of his own house while chasing him with a knife for his infidelity. We made up the next day.

I couldn't understand why I wasn't enough. Why wouldn't he fight to keep our relationship? Why was he interested in other girls? What did those girls have that I lacked? Why didn't he love me enough? Why wasn't I worth enough? The questions played on an endless loop through my head, getting louder and louder. I had no insight into my feelings. I was ramped up on teenage hormones, Depo-Provera, and riding that borderline train into crazy town. My mind was always racing, and my insides were screaming as if tearing through my skin. This was my everyday out-of-control feeling.

Along came Brenna. Chuck and Brenna dated a week, but she would impact my life for a longer period than that. Brenna was enrolled in our high school for precisely three days. She arrived with her bright green hair and glittery black lipstick. Her piercings were flawless, and she had a crazy big chain for her wallet. The school confiscated her chain since it was considered a weapon. She would reach into her bag of tricks and pull out another chain. After the third confiscation, I think the school gave up enforcing the chain rule with her. But that was Brenna. She did what she wanted, and I hated her because she had Chuck. I also secretly admired her.

I started following Brenna in the school halls. I imagined stabbing her with an air-filled syringe, killing her. I would walk so carefully behind her learning her schedule. I was intrigued. What did he see in her? What was she interested in? Then an odd occurrence happened. A common friend informed me that she had stood up for me against Chuck. Chuck had been telling her how "crazy" I was and how she should watch out for me. She had countered with how he should be kind to his ex. She knew about the pain of relationships and stated how my pain and my crazy was probably caused by the head games Chuck was playing. A current girlfriend was standing up for me! This was unheard of. This confirmed it: I wanted to meet her. I had our mutual friend set up a meeting. We ended up hanging out for seventy-two hours straight, and that was the end of her and Chuck. It was also the beginning of Brenna and me.

Brenna was not like my other friends. She was the first of my friends to come from a home that had no rules. A truly dysfunctional home. She ran her own schedule and did what she wanted. Laura had taught me social skills, Chuck had shown me love, but Brenna would teach me survival. The skills of a hustler were more valuable in my life than book smarts.

After-school jobs were for suckers with no vision. I was about to be taken to class for hustlers. She pointed out that I could steal beer and cigarettes from my grocery store job and sell them. I would load up an empty box full of beer, then place the empty box on top while carrying them outside to my car. My job believed I was carrying empty boxes to the dumpster.

I learned about obtaining tests from students in previous quarters. Some teachers didn't change their exams, and now I was selling exams. I made a doctor's office stamp in my graphic arts class. I would use the school pay phone, call myself out as a parent, then stamp myself back in. This was counted as an excused absence and ensured no call home. For a price, I offered my excused absence service. I was now free. Since I could have graduated at sixteen, my senior year consisted of four study halls. I had taken almost all the classes available and had ample free time. Now I was making money and had all the free time to hang out with Brenna. After three days she dropped out of school, but this didn't hinder us from spending time together.

∽

Struggling to maintain my status as Chuck's girlfriend, it would be Brenna that would give me my next identity. This next status would follow me for a few years. My new title was to be a homeless, street-racing drug dealer. But first, I had to graduate high school. College was never an option thanks to my father.

The most frequent question I receive about my life is, "Where was your father?" People often hear stories about my mother and brother, but rarely about my father. I guess there isn't entertainment in telling stories about someone who was as involved as a lamp. The lamp in the room sees all the arguing and yelling. The lamp witnesses the unhappiness, but it has no opinion. My father was an auto factory worker. He worked all day and when he came home, he just wanted to be greeted with dinner. My mother would always have it waiting for him. He wanted the house quiet while he ate so he could watch his nightly TV show, *M.A.S.H.*

I would walk in the door with blood all down the front of my shirt. I would show my father the blood as a result of my mother slapping me. He would look at her and she would say how it's the result of me not eating healthy. I would counter with how it's the result of her slapping me and how it has nothing to do with diet. He would glance at both of us and turn back to the TV. This apparently was not the life he had signed up for.

One perfect night out at a restaurant, I got to see my father lose his stone face. Mother was once again pushing for them to have an anniversary party with a vow renewal ceremony. It was the current trend among their friends. Pushing and pushing, he finally snapped. Right as the server appeared, he yelled, "I don't want to, because if I had to do it all over again, I wouldn't have married you!" Mother burst into tears while the rest of us ordered ice cream without missing a beat. She sulked as she drank her water. No one cared. It was the precise moment we all realized that no one wanted to be in this family.

Which is worse, the direct sabotage from my mother's evil intent or the indirect sabotage from my father's lack of caring? Both yielded to their own destruction. I had the intention to hit the ground running on my adult life. I had traded in my grocery store job for a retail job. I was now using my retail job discount on purchases for my future apartment. I was driving around with a box of brand-new dishes in my trunk. I was seventeen and already packing up my stuff to leave home. I had plans to go to culinary school in Pittsburgh. All I needed was the parental information for my FASFA form.

"It's none of their damn business."

Those were the words that altered my future. Forever those words will be seared into my brain. In that second my whole future went up in flames. I had brought my FASFA forms to my father to apply for financial aid. I just needed his income and other necessary information. With those words, my FASFA was shut down. There was no way for me to receive financial aid without that information unless I applied for emancipation. That also was out of my financial reach. My parents were willing to call in politicians to get my brother pushed through into the military. A simple four-question section was too much for them to bother with for their daughter. My mother's response was that I didn't need to go to college. She stated that instead I just needed to find a man to marry. And just like that, I decided to become a stripper.

This is a perfect example of how people with Borderline Personality Disorder don't see shades of grey. I'm aware of the cliché of a girl becoming a stripper due to not getting love from her father. Although that was true in my case, this was more of a borderline choice. If I could not become a successful college student, a natural next step in life, then I would go to the other side of the spectrum. There is no middle compromise in the borderline mind. Reasonable people might have just moved out and saved up money for school to enroll later. The borderline mind shifts from one extreme to another. If I could not excel and do the traditional option, then instead I would fall into what was considered the dregs of society. The failures of life were to be my friends, and I would attend the school of hard knocks.

Time inched forward toward my high school graduation. And slowly every day I packed another box of belongings. It was a constant two steps forward, one step back situation. My mother had taken to unpacking my belongings some days and arguing about what I was taking with me all days. She would laugh and say I would fail at life if I left home. Confident that I would be unable to support myself, she would constantly say how I was "going to end up dead in a gutter." My standard response was to remind her how being dead in a gutter was better than living a life within these walls.

Graduation day held little happiness. Anytime we had to do an event as a family, it always was just a day of fighting. The only piece of happiness I had was that both Chuck and Brenna were coming to my graduation. The three of us now regularly spent time together. I had to sneak away from my family to thank them for coming. The three of us were all hugging and laughing in a bathroom celebrating my being one step closer to leaving home. It brought me comfort to know somewhere in the large mass of people there were actually two people that cared.

Graduation only made my mother more curious about my plans for providing for myself. I finally informed her that I planned on being a stripper. It was the one job that I knew made enough money to support myself. She reveled in this new-found tidbit of information. She would talk about how men were just going to paw at me and grab me while passing me around. I honestly think that's what she wanted to happen to me. She adored playing a martyr more than any other role.

Considering stress opens the body up to illness, it's no wonder I woke up sick during this time. My fever had spiked, and I couldn't think clearly. I asked my mother to take me to the hospital or urgent care. She refused to take me unless I would take off my black combat boots and put on more "appropriate" shoes. I could not fathom how my fashion taste impacted my need for medical attention. My preference for black clothing was also blamed for why I was feverish.

At this point I realized I was not going to get the medical help I needed from my mother. Here we were again, battling over healthcare. Munchausen by Proxy isn't just the act of making someone sick. It also includes denying them medical treatment. The only medicine I was offered was leftover expired veterinary medication prescribed for Mother's dog. Instead I turned once again to my friends for help.

Being actively involved with school extracurriculars,

I had made a few friends that I could turn to. Leah was on the same dance squad I was, and I knew my parents were unaware of where she lived. Feeling safe about the location, I drove to her house with a fever. I knew my mother would look for me at Brenna's home, so it was not an option. I still parked my car one block over from Leah's house just in case.

Once the car was parked, I began to walk to Leah's. Again, since I had a fever I was disorientated. I walked four blocks in the rain before realizing that I walked the wrong direction and had to turn around. To this day, it is still one of the hardest walks that I ever had to make. Finally, I made it there and she was able to sneak me into her parents' house. It was close to 1 a.m., so it was an easier choice than explaining to her sleeping parents what was going on. Some people don't see the halos they have above their head. That night Leah was indeed my angel. She stayed up all night, bringing me fluids, wrapping me in blankets, and putting cold compresses on my head. She broke my fever of 104. The next day my friends called a meeting to discuss my current situation.

My parents always believed other kids' parents liked them. I can't imagine why they thought that. Mother often commented about how kids never spent time at our house like I spent at others. My friends' parents had met her and wanted their kids around her as little as possible. Mother never knew how many times other parents would hide me and my car from her. They had met my mother and her crazy shined right through. It was to other parents that I would cry about my future as a stripper. They knew I didn't want that. I wanted culinary school. But above that, what I wanted most was to get out of that house.

The meeting took place at Jen's house. Jen was an academically advanced classmate. She was the student that parents encouraged their children to spend time with. Her academics were always on track, so having a meeting at her house was perfect. No parents would suspect any dysfunctional talks occurring at her residence. Leah, Brenna, and Jen sat in a circle around me as I cried. I cried about my future. I cried about how much I was tired of being hit. Both Jen and Leah came from healthy, functional homes. Their optimistic hearts wanted to believe that somewhere deep inside my mother loved me and things could be worked out. Leah was still angry about my mother not helping me when I was sick. She also believed that at the end of the day, a parent loves their child on some fundamental level. Jen was more practical in the viewpoint that there was only a short time left till I turned eighteen and could leave home, so I could just ride it out.

Brenna held a different viewpoint. She was confused by Jen and Leah and did not agree with either. Brenna looked me point blank in the face and said, "She has no right to slap you around. The next time she does that, I would hit her back." All the oxygen in our little circle got inhaled and suddenly all eyes were on me. The idea of hitting a parent never crossed Jen or Leah's mind, or mine in fact. The idea was fascinating. But in that second, my tears stopped, and I realized Brenna was right. I went home that day for the last time.

It was a typical day of Mother ranting about my future as a whore and how I was worthless. Whenever she would start in on me, I would just start packing. It was my go-to passive aggressive move. As she went on and on about my being a whore, I could feel my limit being reached. I spit out the insult of her just being jealous that she's so frigid that father wouldn't touch her. Then the standard crack sound from her slap rang out in my room. This time my head whipped back around to lock eyes. I informed her that if she hit me again then I would hit back. She asked if I thought I was "all that now." My reply was, "I'm all that and a bag of chips." Down came her hand again across my face. I attacked with all the fires of hell consuming me.

I grabbed a fistful of hair on the back of her head and brought her face to my raised knee. As her head came back up, I shoved it further back, slamming it into my bedroom door. A couple of punches to the gut, and she dropped to the floor. And just like that, David slew Goliath. I quickly grabbed my stuff and started loading up my car. In a frenzy, I ripped clothes out of my closet and tossed them in my car. I even grabbed some Chef Boyardee canned ravioli from the kitchen cabinet. As I grabbed the last box, my mother looked up at me, crying. She had remained on the floor while I packed.

I paused to see what she would say. Would she be sorry? Would she apologize? Would she want to talk it out? Her words to me were, "Are you on drugs?" I couldn't even believe that her mind had gone there. I looked down at her red puffy face and said, "Do you think I need drugs to beat you up?" I walked right out the door to start living in my two-door hatchback. My brother would contact me later to laugh and congratulate me on beating up Mother. I had a pager at the time that still allowed people to reach me. He told me how when he came home that day, both parents sat him down. They informed him how he may hear stories from his sister, but nothing I say is true. He asked, "What happened to mother's face?" Father informed him nothing was wrong with her face, and NOTHING happened today. The joys of gaslighting continued. My brother told me how her jaw was swollen and her face was all puffy. He was not allowed to discuss it or acknowledge it.

My brother may have been enjoying their misery, but they were no longer my concern. Living on the streets was now my current situation, and I still wasn't eighteen. Were my parents going to call the cops? It was always a concern. Maybe they didn't because they were worried about a scandal. Or perhaps it was because my mother was afraid to have me back in the house. Either way, I was out of the house.

Brenna started her schooling program of street smarts 101. She got me a wind-up alarm clock to put on the dashboard of my car. This allowed me to wake up to still go to work. I still had the retail job that I was trying to keep. I learned how I could use gas station bathrooms to freshen up as much as possible. I even dyed my hair in a Steak n Shake bathroom. Friends dyed their hair with me to make it more fun. The server came to our table and was like, "Weren't you all different hair colors before?? For a homeless person, I was having a lot of fun. Sometimes Brenna or Chuck would sleep over in my car with me. It was like never-ending car camping.

I learned it was safer to sleep in my car when it was parked in a retirement community. There wasn't a lot of activity there. Police patrolled neighborhoods and parks, so both of those ran risks. People rarely check on the elderly or visit them. Some of them would randomly let me in to use their phone to answer calls to my pager. The retirees didn't care that I was a complete stranger. One lady was so lonely she made me breakfast while letting me use her old-school rotary phone. Most of them were hard of hearing. Brenna and I would hang out on the hood of my car, but they never heard our late-night laughing and talking.

Being homeless was one of the best times for me. There were no schedules, no responsibilities. I could keep whatever hours and go wherever. I was living a carefree, gypsy lifestyle full of complete freedom. If I had lived in a state that was warm year round, I don't know if I would have ever stopped living in my car.

I had learned how to keep myself safe and police free, but I still needed to learn how to survive. Working a part-time retail job was not helping financially. I still wasn't eighteen, so job options were limited. Brenna taught me how to shoplift food ensuring that I wouldn't go hungry. She explained how businesses have insurance to make up for the loss, so it was okay. I learned to only take what I needed, and how it was never acceptable to steal from people, even the people you don't like. I learned about store return policies, such as limits allowed without receipts. This method allowed for stolen goods to be returned for cash. Things like gasoline required cash.

Summer weather cooled as the fall weather rolled in. This marked the arrival of my eighteenth birthday. A new level of freedom entered along with a new set of responsibilities. Mother contacted me and offered her version of a peace offering. She wanted to throw me a birthday party. I declined because I hated her parties. She always just made them about her. I could step away from those parties and not even be missed. She brought up how I had to come by because they wanted to transfer the car title to my name since I was now eighteen. That offer did bring me back to the house.

I hadn't seen my parents since I left. One would think this would be the time they would reach out and try to mend bridges. But this was my family and we only set fire to bridges, usually while someone was standing on it. I met my mother at the license bureau. Since the offer of the car was what I was interested in, I agreed to meet her in public. She always behaved in public and if she was genuine, then she would have no problem meeting me at the license bureau. Everything went smoothly, and she asked if I would come to the house for a visit and catch up. It was such a kind face. I agreed.

I wasn't even there five minutes before a fight broke out. The cake my mother ordered for me was thrown on the kitchen table. She was livid about the fact I refused to be involved with a birthday party. What was there to celebrate? I was homeless. With car title in hand, I left again. I often stayed at Chuck's house under his parents' condition that I slept in his sister's room. It was nice to be able to stretch out on in a bed and take a hot shower. However, this only gave me and Chuck new things to argue about on top of our currently toxic relationship. I would wait all day for him to come home from school because he still had another year of high school left. He would go out with his friends and it would ignite my codependent abandonment issues. It always felt like I was a dog left at home, waiting for someone to come home and give me attention. The constant fighting resulted in me leaving and going back to living in my car.

Now that I was eighteen, I could audition to be a stripper. Finally, I thought I was on my way to securing funds to correct my current living situation. I bought a skimpy silver sequin number, and off to the club I went. The dancers welcomed me with open arms. I hadn't even auditioned yet, but they were giving me recommendations on where to shop for clothes, which clients paid car payments, and roommate suggestions. They all frantically rummaged through their stuff to help me get set up for my audition. One would loan me clothing tape so there was no wardrobe malfunction, while another would lend me a leg garter. The group decided together that my stage name would be Jasmine. Jasmine then took to the stage.

I danced for two numbers. One song I chose was an industrial music track by Nine Inch Nails called "God Money." The lyrics and music screamed as I walked on the stage. I was fascinated to see myself on so many televisions. I was also surprised that so many people visit a strip club during the day. The two songs seemed to take forever, and I left with a fistful of dollars. I got offered the job but declined. It occurred to me that it would be easier to rob the guys in the parking lot than to patiently wait for them to hand over a dollar. My anger level was not a becoming trait in a stripper. I would cycle through a lot of jobs in my life. No new job welcome was ever as kind as the one I received from the group of exotic dancers.

Snow had fallen, and my retail job fired me. I had been calling off a lot because I just didn't care to deal with the people at the job. I was more interested in drinking all night with Brenna and going to concerts. Since I wasn't going to be an exotic dancer, I decided to be a cashier at a gas station. This would reduce one of my bills since I could regularly fill up my car with gasoline for free. I would just fill out drive-off reports saying other random vehicles had filled up and left without paying.

Even with snow, it never occurred to me that living in my car was a problem. I would wake up cold in the middle of the night. After a few minutes of starting up my car heater, my car would be warm enough for me to go back to sleep. One night my friend Nickie came looking for me and had to brush the snow off my windows to see if I was inside. She would later tell me how she honestly thought I was dead. When I asked her for a blanket, she brought me inside her parents' house to live.

Nickie's mom, Mary, had been friends with my mom. She knew through Nickie that I regularly fought with my mother but didn't understand the true extent of it. She witnessed my mother's true colors when she agreed to let me stay at her house. My mother screamed at Mary, demanding that I be thrown back out on the streets. Mary tried explaining to Mother that she should be concerned her own daughter was sleeping outside in the snow. Mother said if Mary didn't throw me out that they would no longer be friends. Mary refused to turn me out into the cold. She explained to my mother that even if she threw me out, I would not return home. She knew I would rather die first.

I wouldn't understand till later in life how much Mary saved me. She fought for a kid that was lost and trying to survive. My friendship with Nickie would last into my adult life. Mary would ask Nickie, whenever she mentioned me, if my mother was still crazy. It became a running joke after how my mother went off on Mary.

I felt safe at Mary's house. I even ordered myself a black futon to sleep on. It was my first piece of furniture! Something as simple as my own futon seemed like such a success. Soon Mary would start asking about how long I intended to stay there. I knew this was not a permanent solution. I also knew my gas station job paid the minimum wage of $5/hr. Hardly enough to move out on. Luckily, I was about to catch a break.

Chuck was now seeing a girl named Kathy. So naturally Brenna and I became friends with her. My routine of befriending his girls to prevent him from dating others never changed. Kathy had been living in a house with her two sisters and was moving out. She arranged for me to meet her sisters Patty and Penny to see about me taking her place in the house. I was given the opportunity to rent the basement for $100/month. This was the break I needed. I moved in my futon and boxes of possessions and put a lock on the door.

The unfinished basement was nothing but a concrete slab with no flooring or carpet. Kathy hung up large pieces of random carpets around a ceiling heat vent to try and trap some heat in a smaller area. I was getting so tired of being cold. Patty never really turned up the heat, so the house was always cold. It was

Cindy Collins

common for people to keep their coats on while there. I eventually went out and bought a space heater for my makeshift room. I had to keep my heater a secret since it ran up the heating bill.

The occupants of the High Street house consisted of Patty, her punk rock husband Nick, and their three-year-old daughter Destiny. The other sister, Penny, was pregnant and lived there with her husband Ben. The house was an odd mix of rednecks drinking Old Milwaukee's Best and punk rockers on LSD. Either way, between the guns and knives within the house, we never had to lock our front door. I was the newest resident in the cockroach-infested drug house. Later, Brenna would join me by squatting on an old child's mattress that was thrown down in the basement as trash.

My functional friends took one look at my newest residence and opted against visiting me at High Street. Their skin would crawl from the poor living conditions. The dead bodies of cockroaches would line the inside door of our microwave. The people they witnessed coming in and out of the house would make them scared of their surroundings. I felt more at home there than I did living with my functional friends. I couldn't breathe in their happy homes with their loving families. All it ever did was amplify how messed up I felt inside. It was if I had "Fucked Up" tattooed on my forehead while around them.

While others would view me as spiraling down, I

viewed it as moving up. I felt so happy about my new place that I even brought in a kitten to be my friend. I would put her in my pocket and drive around with her. She loved climbing all over my makeshift carpet walls. I named her Chlamydia. Chlamydia sounded like a beautiful word to me despite its meaning. I would call her Mydia for short. My friends would call her The Clap for jest. So there I was, living in a drug house with a cat named Chlamydia. Then along came my brother.

While I was graduating high school, my brother had graduated from his career as a burglar, upgrading to a drug dealer. He was still trying to impress others and failing. He would bring over cocaine to my house to be broken down. No one was interested in his coke. His access to LSD was a different story. The standard dose of acid cost $5, so he would sell it for $6 each. Brenna and I would turn around and sell it for $12. He really was the worst criminal on all levels.

As an eighteen-year-old, I now had the opportunity to obtain credit cards. I would cash advance thousands to buy sheets of LSD to turn around and sell for profit. Brenna and I were now constantly on acid. No longer could you see anything in my eyes but dilated black pools. LSD amplified everything I felt and made me super aware of my feelings and surroundings. I never felt so comfortable, so alive. My body was finally in tune with my brain. They were careening through this life at max speed together. The only thing I was missing as a drug dealer was muscle. I was soon transferred to a new gas station job location. In one day walked Billy. He was just what Brenna and I had been missing.

Billy walked into my gas station like a breath of fresh air. His hair was in a mohawk while wearing an obscure band T-shirt. I had spray painted the portrait of the band's lead singer on the hood of my car. That sealed our friendship. Billy was a skater kid who had heart for days. Although his heart for his friends was never-ending, he came with a bite. He had been chasing his mom's abusive boyfriends out of the house since the age of eleven. He couldn't count how many skateboards he had broken over classmates' heads in school. Like me, he would laugh and have fun but could turn in a second. The rapid flip in emotions is a common defense mechanism in anyone that has endured trauma. In Billy, I finally found the brother I had always wanted. Billy was my protector.

If Billy was the muscle, then Brenna was the voice of reason. When out at a 24-hour diner with friends, we would all go around the table sharing our number of sexual partners. Chuck disclosed his number, which didn't add up with the total I had been told. Everyone's head looked down in embarrassment. It clicked that everyone had known about his cheating and he didn't even care to hide it by lying about his number.

It took a split second for my hand to reach the knife on the table. Before I could plunge it into Chuck, Brenna's hand had smacked down on mine as fast as I had hit that knife. Barely audibly, she growled the words "Not... here . . ." There is no fuse for those with Borderline Personality Disorder, no thoughts of consequences. A person with Borderline Personality Disorder has less impulse control receptors in their brain compared to others who do not have Borderline Personality Disorder. Reaction to an emotion is always fast and extreme. Brenna had learned to react and anticipate my reactions to navigate me through. I had zero healthy coping skills.

On the car ride home with Chuck and his friend, I got out of the car and opted to walk home in the snow. I couldn't breathe in that environment; I couldn't continue being in a situation where I wasn't able to react. Brenna also got out and joined me for the two-mile walk home back to High Street at one in the morning. She got me laughing by making fun of how we were both a couple of "dumb bitches" for shaving our heads in the winter. It was just my luck that it started to snow for our walk home. Once again, I was cold.

The majority of nights would start with me and Brenna donning our spiked jewelry and combat boots with fishnet stockings and packing up LSD to unload. Sometimes I would sell the LSD out of my gas station. I would keep it in Tupperware and store it in the store ice bin. Cops would come in and lean up on the ice bin while drinking the store coffee for free. It always made me secretly smile.

We could run the night without a care in the world,

knowing that no one could touch us. The punks in the house were using mop handles to teach us how to spar and fight. Between being armed with a tire iron and traveling with Billy, I never felt safer. It was nothing for me to walk into a store with a tire iron and threaten someone at their job for money owed. One store overcharged my friend $7. He called out the clerk, and the clerk said it was he said/she said, and there was nothing my friend could do about it. I went in with a tire iron and got the $7 back along with another store ban. Only in a truly violent environment did I find safety and comfort. The chaos was so similar to my home environment that it felt natural.

The incident that cemented our little trio's reputation was the day someone stole $20 from me. Billy invited him to the self-serve car wash to buy some drugs. When the kid arrived, Billy pulled down the door to the car wash stall. All the people in the other stalls could hear the screams. Everyone scattered before the police arrived. The cherry on the sundae was for a week after that, Billy called and played the song "Working at the Car Wash" on the kid's answering machine. Being violent was one thing, but rubbing salt in the kid's wounds for additional torture showed a darker side. I finally had power to wield, power that I had desired for my whole life. However, I never asked Billy for his "services." I loved him too much to deliberately put him in extreme danger. The piece of family he offered me mattered more than any life he could have executed. To us, it was never about the $20 or even the $7. It was about respect and taking care of our friends. Respect was what we had never received in life. Respect was what we were now taking.

Drug money was substantial, and I could make it rain free drugs on all my friends. Late at night we would all go to an all-night retail store on LSD. We would ride display bikes around the store, throw bowling balls down aisles, and load cassette tapes in store display radios, among other chaotic things. Billy taught me how to skateboard in a store. He popped open a new skateboard, threw it down on the linoleum, and gave me tips as I skated through the aisles at 3 a.m. The world was our playground. The borderline was happy.

The happiness from drugs paled in comparison to the euphoria I felt when street racing. They say borderlines are known for extreme behavior such as excessive drug use, drinking, or driving recklessly. The borderline in me was definitely in charge during this time period. On an average day, I would never stop for stop signs and would barely break for red lights. It was a combination of believing I was going fast enough that I couldn't be hit and a bit of just not caring. I was constantly pushing my limits just to feel alive or feel anything but the deadness I felt inside. Of all the drugs I would try, adrenaline was still my favorite.

Brenna and I would pick racing targets based on car decals. Trucks with male machismo stickers were more likely to accept racing for money. That type of men always thought it was cute to race girls. When they lost, they would try to flirt their way out of paying the money owed. That was when Billy would get out of the car and collect.

I had been racing since high school. I didn't start racing cops or racing for cash until later when fueled by drugs. But every day after school, I would race the same kid down the same roads. He was always salty when he would lose. I think that's why he would push for me to take the oncoming lane of traffic during the race. I would jump curbs and cut through yards when necessary. I had already become comfortable with the idea of dying. Before passengers entered my car I gave a disclaimer that there was a potential of impending death. The other fun rule of riding in my car was girls always get shotgun... even if a guy calls it first.

Later, on acid, I would have drug kids jump out of my car while it was moving. I would have to turn the car around to make sure they were okay. I had people get out at random places, lie about how they knew someone there, and ask me to continue my night without them. Being a passenger in my vehicle was not for the weak of heart. Nothing about my lifestyle was for the weak. Ironically those who were weak and preyed on by life were now rising up with the strength of a phoenix. Blazing paths of fire and vengeance was my nightly release.

Cash was coming in from drugs and now from street racing. Minimum-wage jobs do not support life.

Thanks to Brenna, I had learned to always be looking for a side hustle for extra income. Society will never admit it, but the truth is that crime does pay. Surprisingly enough, stalking is a lucrative side hustle. Long before checking into places on Facebook, people had no idea where others were located. It seemed that men were always going to cheat, and girls always wanted to catch them. Therefore, tracking down girls' boyfriends was a plentiful and profitable night's work.

Brenna and I would get a multi-city map and a highlighter and plan our route for the night. We would make sure all the men were where they were supposed to be. If there were any random cars at their house, then the license plate, make, and model was reported back. Considering we could go days with no sleep on acid, we had tons of time to track people down. I always preferred to keep Brenna in the car with me. Stalking people on my own always made me feel crazy. If I had a friend in the car, then it was just seen as a crazy night of work filled with drug-fueled shenanigans.

My stalking skills and tracking people down had long ago been perfected by keeping tabs on Chuck. I would spend hours on acid sitting outside his house in my car, waiting for him to get home just to see who he had been spending his time with. It was during this time that Chuck joined the military and left the state. My friends always joked with me saying he did that because it was the only way he could finally date other girls. I would laugh on the outside with others. Inside I felt my self-hatred grow. My crazy actions had ruined the relationship.

Would I ever be able to count on someone for love? I felt so unworthy of love. Sometimes I would discuss going to California to find him. It truly felt that he was the only person in the world who could love me. The joyous black and white thinking of a borderline. Brenna would feed me LSD to distract me from my thoughts ramping up and spiraling out of control.

I had traded a hectic school schedule for a hectic hustler schedule. At least I now had drugs to keep up with things. My brain was always pushing me forward, speeding out of control. The chaos was still more comfortable to deal with than being alone in my thoughts. That is when the suicidal thoughts were the loudest. Most mornings by this point had me waking up angry and disappointed to be alive. How was I surviving this life? I felt so weak because I couldn't go through with ending my life myself. But I couldn't understand how I was surviving with the amount of drugs I was consuming. My body was refusing to overdose. The same could not be said for my friends.

The party was about to come to an end. Once again, my brother was arrested. I usually couldn't care less when he went to jail. Except for this time, he was my access to LSD. His arrest hurt me financially. This time he broke into a junior high while high on cocaine. He had safecracking tools, drugs, and a gun on him. I guess he was planning on stealing kids' lunch money?

Apparently, he was unaware of a thing called daily night deposits. Resisting arrest was another charge added that ensured he went to big boy prison for the first time. County jail, where Mother watched over him, was not an option. I will say it again: worst criminal ever.

Sobriety was not an option. I went with my parents to visit my brother in prison, hopeful he would give me a contact name that could assist me with my supply needs. The visit was pure dysfunction. My father sat there in silence, refusing to speak to anyone. I couldn't tell if this was a normal day for him or if he was upset with the situation. My drama queen of a mother just sat there crying. She would complain of the long drive and having to buy a clear purse to get through security. I would wink and smile at prisoners in the yard behind the glass just to antagonize my mother. My brother would comment that a few murder one prisoners were in his cell block. I could pick out every single one of them. What can I say? My taste in men is impeccable.

Side conversation with my brother consisted of him asking me to send him money, LSD, and a gold chain, and to work with Billy on breaking him out of prison. I informed him that I had zero money for him and considering acid amplifies your feelings, I don't think prison is where I would want to be hallucinating. Also, a gold chain was not going to help his scrawny ass fit in, and it would just be taken. And when did Billy gain prison-breaking skills? He had no idea what he truly needed in there to survive. I told him to make a big friend. I did find it ironic that he was about to learn what it was to be passed around. Karma may be a bitch, but she was only showing me her sweet side.

With my brother gone that put me back on mother's radar. Suddenly she was blowing up my pager wanting me to come over. When she did convince me to visit, all she wanted to do was discuss my brother and the tragedy of his being locked up. Here we are once again expected to feel sorry for those that are responsible for ruining their own lives. My brother would admit that he was high at the time of the crime. He would admit that he was doing the job for money for drugs. Never once did he admit he was a junkie. He always wrongly thought he had everything under control. With drugs, there is no control.

Fired from my gas station job for attendance call offs, I was out of work. Living off credit cards seemed fine. At nineteen years old, I was finally able to secure a job in a furniture warehouse. I would work as both a call center worker and a switchboard operator. I would turn off the switchboard to have the incoming call beep throughout the warehouse. That way I could hang out in the break room with the drivers playing cards. If a call came in, I could just transfer it from the breakroom phone to wherever it needed to go. Always angling for a side hustle, it wasn't long before I was making extra cash gambling with the drivers.

Some days I would turn down the volume on the switchboard so people couldn't hear it beep. If they walked by my desk, they couldn't hear calls waiting. They presumed I was in the bathroom. In reality, I was out hanging out with friends or grocery shopping. The whole warehouse crew was a certain level of dysfunction. How did I always fall into these environments?

The drivers would carve out holes in store mattresses to hold their liquor battles. They would drink, pass out, and take a nap during their shifts. It was no big deal for me to sleep at work after a late night at the club. I would come dressed in black vinyl spiked-out club gear from the previous night and pass out on the floor. Some coworkers would meet up and have sex on the same mattresses that we would sell to customers. This was my new job.

Billy would sometimes visit me at work. We would have office chair races with other people. I would sit Indian style in the chair while Billy would push me while running. Other days we would play roller ball in the warehouse on roller blades. I loved the playful side of Billy more than his violent side. It should be no surprise that eventually the furniture business went bankrupt.

The warehouse would be my introduction to office politics. People with Borderline Personality Disorder often change jobs or get fired. We lack healthy conflict resolution skills and are not skilled at engaging with people. Anytime you deal with people, there is some level of compromise to be learned. Compromise requires seeing a middle, a grey part. That part did not exist within me. I ran my call center the way I ran the streets, with fear and violence.

Surprisingly, my mania and rapid-firing problem-solving skills make me an efficient employee. Only seeing black and white means that I follow rulebooks to the letter. However, when that emotional side gets triggered, the rule book is burned. Also, I lack regular attendance skills since having the same daily routine makes me feel trapped. Knowing my attendance is weak, I would eventually learn how to navigate company attendance policies.

Days would go by in the warehouse, and I would answer numerous calls with no issue. The moment a customer would try and shred me, things would change. I would answer back to the customer that they should rethink how they talk to people, people who had access to their address. The phone line would always immediately go dead quiet with shock. Threatening customers or coworkers was no different to me than threatening someone who owed me money for drugs.

Coworkers always thought the way I pushed back on customers was hilarious. They quickly learned that it wasn't so funny when my anger was directed at them. I walked over to a station and hung up a girl's phone while she was mid-conversation. I told her how I was tired of picking up her slack, and it was already explained she made too many personal calls. When she pushed back, I offered to meet her in the parking lot after work. She was about seven months pregnant. I told her how I had no problem hitting her so hard that her child would be born bruised. The drivers later came out to the parking lot to take wagers on who would win the fight. The girl never showed that night. She also never came back to work.

Managers loved how efficient I was but also learned how difficult I could be. Three managers sat me down in the break room. Without a word, they slid a piece of paper toward me. They waited while I read my write-up. I stood up, not breaking eye contact with them, and tore the piece of paper slowly in half. After I threw the shredded paper in the air, I walked out. Later people would tell me how they overhead the managers say, "That went better than I thought it would."

Adapting or learning from incidents like that was never an option. It always seemed to make my fiery hate burn brighter. The joy of being subjected to trauma is your feelings are constantly thrown off by the hormones created from your sympathetic nervous system. This meant my only options at work were fight or flight. I would either come back with the handbook, fueled by adrenaline, trying to argue how wrong they were, or I would just quit. I couldn't even count how many jobs I have had in this lifetime.

The drug scene seemed easier to navigate than the job market. My current scene was falling apart. I had lost my drug supply, and now I was losing my friends. One might think they were drug friends, so they left when the drugs did. That was not true. Drugs were the reason they indeed did leave me. One by one, my friends started to die from overdosing. Others went to prison. Slowly I was losing my chaotic scene that had brought me comfort. Their lost smiling faces would haunt me for years. I would remember them riding bikes around a store at 3 a.m. At least I still had the cat.

Billy was now running with a full-blown FBI-wanted gang. He was flying to different states to "take care" of situations. It seemed like with every job he did with his new group, a piece of the Billy I knew would die. He was losing his playful, carefree side and turning darker. Brenna relocated to a city an hour away to move into her own party house. She was joining the rave scene since she now was mainlining crystal meth. My own version of family was leaving me. I decided to move to the city Brenna was living in. Apartments there would not approve my application since I didn't have a local job or meet their income requirements. I was trying so hard to cling to this life, for it was my identity. Who was I without Brenna and Billy? Following Billy into his gang did not appeal to me, which left Brenna for me to follow. An average person might have just applied to jobs in that area, or maybe applied to an apartment with different income requirements. But I was a borderline with no coping skills. On the opposite side of the spectrum, I jumped.

Without acid I was in search of a new reckless high. Searching for something to appease the borderline in me. People often talk about how borderlines abuse drinking and drugs. Other characteristics that are rarely mentioned is reckless unsafe sex with people and excessive spending. I traveled in the social circle of punks. Punks aren't really sexual people. Their "go to" action is usually violence, so the act of sex seems to confuse them. It looked like spending was to be my next high.

If I couldn't afford an apartment, then I would buy a car. Not just a used car but a brand-new cherry red car. I was nineteen years old and buying a brand-new car. The dealership was running a special. If I purchased brand new, then they would throw in a prepaid $400 gas card. I could use some free gas in my life. I chose all the bells and whistles. I even opted for a moon roof on the car. I almost opted for a convertible. I decided against that for fear of strangers randomly jumping in my car. The car was so beautiful that none of my friends could believe that I didn't steal it. It was easy to understand since I had a history of criminal activity. Assuming it was stolen, they refused to let me park my car in front of their houses.

So, I'm in trouble at my job, my friends are scattering, I have a large car payment, credit card debt, and still can't afford a decent apartment. The logical thing in my mind was to take the gas card and head to New York City. I decided to pick up Brenna along the way for the road trip. I just had to check her out of the hospital first. When I would make plans in my head and incorporate people, it was never an option to me that they wouldn't comply. No matter the circumstances, I would make things happen.

Brenna had just undergone an appendectomy. She now had a boyfriend who was ultimately against me taking her to New York. She hadn't been out of the hospital twelve hours. I pinned her guy flat on the ground with my tire iron against his throat while Brenna packed her bags. Even in her drugged-up haze and leftover surgical pain, she wasn't going to pass on a free trip to New York.

In true borderline fashion, I set the cruise control on the car at 105 mph, and we were off to New York. Driving late at night, I expected that the only other vehicles on the road would be drunks or police. We had no intentions at stopping for either. One cop in New Jersey did attempt to pull us over. The rate of speed gave us such a head start that we were able to get off a random exit ramp and lose him. Back on the road we went with our cruise control engaged.

The Tibetan Freedom Festival was a two-day outdoor music festival. The proceeds of the event went to support Tibet's freedom from the Chinese dictatorship. By supporting Tibet, you are entered on a list that is not allowed in China. I gladly signed away my rights to visit China in exchange for a weekend of punk rock music. Nights were spent walking the streets of downtown to see the sights. In one of the biggest cities, I still wasn't scared of potential crime or violence. The violence I witnessed in New York made me question my current path.

In New York, I would see people get mugged and scream for help. The police would sit and drink their coffee while watching the criminal run by. Traffic lights, speed signs, and driving rules were optional. I felt like I had been training for driving in downtown New York my whole life. New York was one big free for all. Was this the life that would be good for me? Brenna already wanted to stay and was pricing apartments. Could I see myself in this life?

My defining New York moment wasn't at Central Park, Rockefeller Center, or the Statue of Liberty. The moment that woke me up was on a random subway platform. I looked over, and standing next to me was a little old lady. She stood there with her purse wide open showing the cash that was inside. I knew I could just grab her purse, push her off the platform, and run. In that second, I realized a shift. I had gone from using little old ladies' phones while chatting over breakfast to thinking about pushing them off subway platforms. How had this happened? How had I gotten so dark and out of control? I knew that living in New York would seal my future by letting me sink lower into that darkness.

I passed on the idea of living there. On the way home, we stopped off at the Hershey, Pennsylvania theme park. We ran around the theme park wearing Hershey kiss beanie hats while gorging on free chocolate bars. The laughter and carefree fun we had while posing for pictures with a huge Rolo candy bar could not have happened if we had stayed in New York. In New York, there would have been no laughing or carefree fun to feed my internal kid. We left the moon roof open for the ride home. The propellers on our hats spun for the remainder of the car ride. Despite all my past, I was still just a lost kid. I was a borderline burning through the world like a supernova.

Living as a Borderline

※

Returning home after New York was like waking up with a hangover. I was suddenly awake and aware of how raw my body was feeling from extended drug use. Slowly my friends were dying from trying more severe drugs. The remainder of my friends were going to jail for turning into junkies. Was this my life? What does a "normal" life look like for a borderline? I didn't know what I wanted. I just knew I wanted something else for myself than my current life. I firmly believe people enter your life to get you through that specific part of life. When I was feeling the lowest, that's when the universe gave me a saint. Saint Greg sent me a letter.

Greg had become my friend when I was fourteen years old and he was seventeen. Shortly after he graduated high school, he joined the army. We would write to each other during his boot camp stay.

Randomly we would keep coming in and out of each other's lives. This time he had just gotten divorced and decided to look me up. He was hoping I wasn't still with Chuck and was available for dating. I couldn't dial his number fast enough. With both feet, the borderline jumped into the next relationship, eager for the next identity.

The night I met with Greg, he gave me a key to his house. I now had my own sanctuary. My own place to hide away from the life that was leaving me with a grimy feel. In about three months, I was completely moved in. I even brought my cat named Chlamydia with me to Greg's. Being with Greg felt easy. We had that solid foundation of friendship. I also felt safe with him. I had known him for years, so I felt secure and protected. Sadly though, being in a relationship amplifies my borderline tendencies. No matter what Greg did, there was no way to have avoided the incoming chaos.

The drugs and criminal activities were all left behind when I started with Greg. It was too awkward to try and explain why I was hiding Billy's blood-soaked car in the garage. I traded in my spikes and combat boots for business suits. I decided that a job as a bank teller would make me more of a respectable girlfriend. However, when your body has been racing a million miles per second, the crashing halt takes its toll. I still had been dealing with my endometriosis pain. Greg encouraged me to go to the doctor to get checked out. Now that I had a better job with insurance, I scheduled the appointment. This would start the never-ending cycle of doctors.

For years my endometriosis had been growing, unchecked. Recent exams showed I also had dysplasia, pre-cancerous cells of the cervix. Cervical cancer is rapid-spreading, so the doctor remained diligent about lasering it off every four to five months. Every few months, I was having outpatient surgery for the dysplasia. Once a year, I would have to be checked into a hospital for treatment of the endometriosis. Greg was there for every single procedure. He would hold my hand while chunks of my cervix would be cut away for lab tests.

Despite all the procedures, my monthly cycle was still excruciating. I wouldn't make it to work when I was menstruating. I would beg Greg to kill me so I wouldn't have to continue with this pain. Doctors would tell me that I should have a child to help cure my endometriosis. That has never made sense to me. Why would I have a child just to help myself? Also, the rate of dysplasia regrowth was a concern. The chance that I could be pregnant for nine months without developing cervical cancer was slim.

Was this my new life? Was my body failing? I blamed myself. I believed that all the hate that I carried somehow rotted away my insides. I was twenty-two years old and was once again angry to be alive. How was I supposed to balance my new banking job with my failing health? The universe tilted again, except this time it dumped my mother on me.

Greg didn't have my new address, so his original letter went to my mother's house. She notified me of it and suddenly became very interested. She viewed Greg as a solid potential future husband for me. She wanted to have the married daughter with kids to help her fit in with her friends. I just never knew the lengths that she would go to try and obtain it.

Borderlines are often accused of being manipulative. It's rarely discussed how easy it is to manipulate someone diagnosed with Borderline Personality Disorder. With no sense of true self and an insatiable thirst for love and acceptance, plus the famous push-pull in relationships, we have buttons to be pushed. It's really very simple to set off a borderline, and my mother excelled at it. I would feel dizzy from being spun around so many times.

The standard fight would be her asking me, "Well, if he loves you, why isn't he asking you to marry him?" Then I would rage on Greg, accusing him of not loving me. It must be so apparent that he doesn't love me since others are bringing it up. Then he would state that he just got out of a marriage and we haven't even been together a year. Rational fights have no place in this situation.

I would go crying back to Mother about how he was refusing to marry me. Then she would state how I was being super insensitive to Greg since he'd just gotten divorced, and I needed to give him more time. Then a week later she would ask me the same question and set me off on Greg again. Was it sport for her? Did she just enjoy pulling my strings and watching me dance? It became so common that before any argument between Greg and me, he would ask if I had talked to my mother that day. He knew I was getting spun around.

I finally had my mother's full attention, and it was breaking me. People always question why I maintained contact with her for so many years. Children still want to believe on some level that their parents love them. For one simple reason, if your parents don't love you, how can anyone else? You are a part of your biological parents. It should be built into them to love you as their child. The concept of a parent not loving their child, only loving to torture them? That's difficult for anyone to understand.

The cycle of spinning me around continued for a while. My family tried to seem like the perfect family to Greg. My parents would be affectionate and make like they were happy when he was around. They would shower presents down on him for the holidays. He would end up with more gifts than me. But the level of crazy my mother contained couldn't be held for long. She would call me out in front of Greg. She would tell Greg how she's on his side and how I just need to be more patient regarding a marriage. Any chance she had to make me look like the crazy one, she took the shot. The gaslighting was turned up to maximum capacity.

Mother would always ask about my health in front

of Greg. She always loved to look like a caring mother. I didn't know until later why she was so interested in my doctors' appointments. In private, she would tell me to have a kid to fix my health. When I told her that I wasn't ready for a child, her response was, "You will get used to it. I did." That cemented my decision to never have children.

Later I learned that mother had also started telling her friends that I had cancer. Dysplasia was pre-cancerous, not cancer, yet my mother was running around with ribbons crying about her daughter having cancer. It took me a moment to catch on to what had been happening behind my back. People were randomly coming up to me congratulating me on "getting out of the house," or I would get people crying tears of joy because they found me in a grocery store buying food. They were cheering about me doing everyday mundane tasks.

While mother was playing town crier about a nonexistent cancer, I was going with Greg to his family's weekly Sunday dinners. In her true competitive nature, mother started inviting us over for dinners. I never got a dinner invite when I was stealing food and homeless, but now that I had a suitable gentleman caller, I had value. I would instruct Greg to follow my lead on what to eat. I had learned to navigate what food was deemed safe. Greg ventured down his own path once. After a night in the bathroom, he never questioned what I said about her food again. He also got in the habit of checking the expiration dates of food she would bring by. She was regularly dropping off expired food at our house. Greg would smile, accept it graciously, and then throw it in the trash.

Dinners at my mother's house consisted of rules and strategy; dinner at Greg's parents was even more difficult for me. Greg had a wonderful, functional family. They didn't just have weekly dinners together because it was required. They did it because they truly loved each other and wanted to spend time with each other. I couldn't fathom this idea of family. I didn't understand going to dinner and not having rules or not having to edit myself. It only amplified my feeling of dysfunction.

I never felt so out of place as I did with Greg's family. They were those rare individuals that are genuinely nice and honestly caring people. I placed so much pressure on myself to fit in and succeed. I was a master at assuming identities since I didn't have one of my own. But how do you assume an identity of a functional family-loving individual? I couldn't even grasp the concept. I couldn't breathe in that environment.

More and more, I was getting immersed in healthy environments. I was training at the credit union to learn to work in other departments and move up into management. I was also spending time at Greg's parents' house and would occasionally go shopping with his mom. Farther and farther away from the streets I traveled. The healthier the situation, the more I struggled.

Mother had gone from spinning me around over marriage to holding up a mirror to the house I was living in. Greg had bought the house with his inheritance money, and it was in his mom's name. I kept getting spun to only see it as the house that he bought his previous wife. It was suddenly as if the house were just scraps thrown to me. *I get to live there, but not as a wife.* Did I even want to get married? That question never entered my mind.

What I wanted more than anything was for everything to stop. I would jump through mother's hoops, not for acceptance but for her silence. I wanted to stop being triggered. It was exhausting, and my body started shutting down. Now I had developed full-blown anxiety attacks. My muscles would tighten up so that I was locked in a fetal position. I would hyperventilate until I passed out. I didn't even link it to the fact that surrounding myself with my family was the same as surrounding myself repeatedly with my sexual assault trauma. I still thought all of this was a normal reaction to stress.

The fighting between Greg and me was increasing. If he offered me a salsa that I didn't like, I would immediately start packing my bags. *How could I marry a man that doesn't know what salsa I like?* Yeah, it ramped up that quick in the mind of a borderline. I would be screaming and packing while he was standing there confused, holding a bag of tortilla chips in his hand.

Greg knew the pressure I was under. I believe that

was factored in when he proposed. It should have been a happy moment, but all I thought was, "Is mother going to complain about how he proposed?" Greg had tried to appease my family. He went so far as to ask my father's permission before asking me. My father told him, "You can do better." That was the day that Greg really started to hate my family. My attempts to explain to Mother that Father's response was inappropriate were countered with accusations of lack of sense of humor. There is nothing funny about putting down your child.

Now that we were engaged, I thought I could just breathe. I believed this would get mother out of my hair, and I could just enjoy being with Greg. Once again, that was not to happen. I explained to mother that I wanted to spend some time just enjoying being engaged. After all, we had still not been dating a year. Mother broke into tears and explained how she was dying. Mother claimed that she had previously had breast cancer. The cancerous part that was cut out left one of her breasts deformed. She tried to correct the shape by getting breast implants. She also stated that my father was embarrassed by her previous breast size, so she increased her size. The implant was now leaking silicone into her bloodstream, slowly killing her. Insurance would not cover the cost to have it removed, so death was inevitable. This was her story. This was the story told and accepted because it was in a pre-Google time frame.

Later in life, articles would be posted proving her to be a liar. Of course, her still being alive would also debunk her lies. The National Center for Health Research would post the following: "Moreover, in one of his papers on the topic, Dr. Blais determines that implants can injure without undergoing mechanical failure. Studies on long-term implant users indicate that, in the pectoral and intercostal areas, gradual and irreversible deterioration of muscle function takes place. Respiratory problems are widespread among implant users, as are complications affecting major lymphatic ducts and fluid irrigation of the upper chest" (Van den Berg, 2018). That explains how later she would develop emphysema and blame my smoker father for it. It seems more likely her breathing problems were brought on by her vanity.

I was going to believe the FDA organization over a woman who believed tampons can only be used by non-virgins. According to WebMD, "In 2006, after reviewing research and finding no connection between silicone gel implants and disease, the FDA approved the sale of certain silicone gel breast implants" (Gardner, 2019). But since Google was not available yet, I cried over my mother dying.

I cried because I wanted more time in hopes that I would finally have the mother-daughter relationship that I had always wanted. Borderlines struggle with abandonment, which they feel more intensely. Losing anyone in your life feels like part of you has died. Loss is the most challenging thing for a borderline, and I was trying to comprehend the loss of a parent.

Mother was now educating me on how to take care of estate planning when she was gone. She would tell me where keys and safe combinations were. She took me to the bank to add me to her safe-deposit box. According to her, a copy of her last will and testament was located inside. The decree would name me the Executor of State, although I have never seen a copy of the will. My brother already had a copy of the will, but she said I didn't need a copy since I was on the safe deposit box. Years later, I would find out that she removed me. I'm guessing that action occurred the day after she added me.

Every night Greg would hold me while I cried for the impending loss. It never occurred to me that her "cancer" was as fake as the cancer she claimed I had. Suddenly in all the sadness, mother suggested that she wanted to see me married before she died. She stated how her imminent death was coming fast. This is how she gained control of my wedding. She had lied and caused grief over an impending fake death, just to have a say over which bakery created my wedding cake.

If you ask any of my friends to describe my wedding to Greg, their response is always, "Oh, you mean Cindy's mom's wedding?" It was the running joke among my friends during this time. Even on my wedding day, my friends toasted to me, "Happy Cindy's mom's wedding day!" During this time, I became very familiar with alcohol. Drinking became the vice that helped me deal with my family. My bridal party would make drinks before any event that involved my mother. They all needed a crutch to deal with her. I would be drunk walking down the aisle. Mother had the wedding of her dreams. She chose the cake from the same bakery that created her wedding cake. I wanted a strawberry cake from another bakery, but that wasn't an option. Sometimes I would secretly visit bakeries and try wedding cakes to imagine what it would be like to pick out my own wedding cake. She picked out the colors, the flowers, the church, and the clergy and even designated herself my matron of honor.

The guest list was over 200 people, and I only knew those that I placed in my bridal party. She stated how it was her turn to get money back. She felt she should be given the money that she had gifted to others' weddings. The guest list was composed of those that she felt owed her. Out of town guests were also a bonus because she thought they would just send a check and she wouldn't have to pay for their headcount at the reception. My wedding generated thousands in cash, not counting gifts. I was to be sold to Greg.

The interesting part of my wedding day is it's the only time my father ever said the words "I love you" to me. Right before walking me down the aisle, he kissed me on the cheek and said those words. But how can a man that never spoke to me or spent time with me love me? Did he love me, or did he love the idea that one of his kids was turning out "normal"? Once again, a marriage to a man gave me value as a person.

Greg and I skipped out on the reception as soon as possible. We went out to eat with our friends for our own personal reception. Before catching our honeymoon flight to the Bahamas, I called my mother to thank her for the lovely wedding. The movie *The Father of the Bride* showed a daughter doing that, so I thought that was how ordinary people behaved. I was still masquerading as an average functional person. When I got back from my honeymoon, my life as a borderline wife would begin.

Considering television was my built-in childhood babysitter, it should come as no surprise that I learned how to be an adult based on movies. When you think normal life is Hollywood movies, that's a standard that no one can achieve. I believed being married was all about group family dinners and events and having adventures with your spouse. No one tells you that the reality is married life is boring, with a typical day-to-day grind. Going from an adrenaline-fueled lifestyle to a calm daily routine was making my insides scream.

I attempted to host co-family meals. My family refused to come to a dinner to which Greg's family was also invited. I would get stressed and overwhelmed, which would end up with me throwing a tray of dinner rolls down the stairs. Nothing was working out as I thought it should. Every move was made in an attempt to silence mother or appease her "dying wish."

Greg agreed to move into a different house. I chose a grander house to show how great at life I was doing. Greg signed off on the mortgage for a home that he hadn't even seen yet. He agreed to anything to keep me happy. Although mother triggered me about living in Greg's first house, she was more upset after I moved. I would then be accused of considering myself a better person because my house was more beautiful than hers. Most parents want their kids to do better than they did. Mine were not in that parental category.

The dying wish card got played out again when she tried to convince me to have children. I told her the death con she had been running was over. She stopped talking about it and moved on. Just like that, mother was well again. Now she would return to her usual game of spin control. I tried to talk to mother about feeling suicidal and struggling with the day to day of married life. Her response was, "It's part of marriage." Next thing I knew, she had given me a gun as a random present. Then she invited Greg and me to join her and my father on vacation. So, was I to commit suicide or go on vacation first, then die? I could never tell up from down.

I was surprised to be invited on vacation. Finally, a real family vacation—or so I thought. When we reached our destination, we rarely saw my parents. They were constantly ditching Greg and me. Greg was livid. He couldn't understand why they would invite us somewhere but not want to spend time with us. Once again, even on a family vacation, I was left behind. At least now I had Greg. We both agreed that "family" vacations like that would never happen again.

Between the mounting pressure of Greg not supporting contact with my family, and me feeling like an outsider to his family, I snapped. During an argument with Mother, I told her I was done with the family and never wanted any contact from any of them again. At first, she sent daily letters filled with hateful speech. I was accused of being the ungrateful daughter that didn't appreciate the kindness she had shown me. Then the letters stopped, or maybe Greg started throwing them away. Either way, suddenly I felt free. I would hide away in my big house with my husband and never have to deal with them again. But Mother's reach was far and wide.

Currently, I was working in the credit union's corporate office in the mail room. I had been on management fast track but scrapped that plan. In one year, I had changed departments three times. With no conflict resolution skills, I was having a difficult time getting along with coworkers. I kept changing departments to avoid being fired.

One average day, a coworker named Brian came into the mail room to show his professional photographer portfolio. Brian worked in asset protection, which meant he monitored potential internal credit union theft. It was a position that highlighted honesty; this looked good on his police academy application. Photography was his hobby. Today when he opened his portfolio, he opened it up to a picture of Mother. Brian was unaware that this was my mother since we now had different last names.

I had known that mother started doing modeling photo shoots a few years prior. It always seemed odd to me. She would bring home clothes that were supposedly gifted to her as a prize or bring home a trophy that she had won from the shoot. The trophies were for weird categories like Best Smile, Best Poses, or Best Outfits. Father would complain that her modeling wasn't paying enough, and she needed a different job. Mother even picked up an agent named Eric. She and Eric would regularly go to lunch. She would have shelves filled with colossal photo albums of pictures of herself. She would carry collections around with her to show to her family members. The living room would have a wall of nothing but images of her. Shelves were built to display her trophies.

I was very interested in learning about these photo shoots from Brian's perspective. He discussed how the model in the picture, my mother, had made him uncomfortable by hitting on him. Brian was my age and happily engaged. Mother had claimed to be the same age as Brian. I asked him if they ever handed out clothes or trophies at these photo shoots. He looked at me with a strange look and firmly said no. He said the models paid the photographers to take their pictures. Then the models were to take the pictures and build a portfolio to find paid work.

His story made sense. Truth is easy to understand. If the story sounds logical and makes sense, then that is how you can tell the truth. What also made sense to me was that during this time mother was responsible for buying trophies for motorcycle bike shows for her club. Father had been receiving trophies for his motorcycle, and Mother is quite competitive. She had the trophy connection and the ability to buy herself trophies. So, the whole time my father was screaming for financial help, mother was paying others to make her feel pretty about herself. It was the equivalent of getting a JC Penney photo session and then walking out calling yourself a supermodel.

Her "modeling" career came to an end at the hands of my father. She was showing him recent pictures taken of her. He exclaimed how the pink lingerie nightie she was wearing was transparent, and she was naked. She tried defending herself, saying it was just the airbrushed effect. My father wasn't buying that the small-town photographers were bothering with airbrushing techniques. He stated he wasn't interested in seeing any more of her pictures, and that was the end of her modeling.

The fun fact of working in the mail room was that some of my coworkers were members of Mother's church. They all learned the same information I did from the moment Brian opened his portfolio. So now they knew that she had hit on a younger gentleman and was seen all over town with an agent for a nonexistent modeling career. Mother had raised me saying friends that were boys weren't allowed to the house because it looked bad to the neighbors. For someone so concerned about my reputation, she had thrown her reputation to the wind.

I can't say that I was terribly surprised at this revelation. I only wondered if she was trying to gaslight everyone else into buying her modeling career or if she believed it herself. Her vanity was always known based on how she would handle charity events. She would spearhead a charity activity, but then call the press out to cover the event. She would clip out the article of herself and create a massive photo album of her works. Are you really doing good deeds if you need to be rewarded and recognized for them? These works would be submitted yearly to nominate herself for the town's hall of fame. Years of campaigning, and she would finally secure her spot in the town's hall of fame.

Haunted. That is the word that describes how I felt. Everywhere I turned, I couldn't shake her. She would be on the news and friends would call me. They would make jokes about how great she looked on TV and how it must be because she was a "model." Everyone would laugh behind her back but never call her crazy out to her face. I didn't even have time to process this information due to the fact I was about to be admitted to the hospital.

I had given up the fight with endometriosis. My

OB/GYN doctor finally agreed to give me a hysterectomy at the age of twenty-three years old. He would tell me later that this surgery saved my life. My ovary was about to burst from inflammation. He also stated that the area underneath my uterus was covered with endometriosis. The yearly surgeries of lasering it off were all for nothing since the majority was inaccessible without uterus removal.

I would always wonder throughout life if I could have avoided a hysterectomy. If I had been brought a doctor instead of cups of hot chocolate, would my fertility have been saved? How would my health situation have been different with a different family? The church members that I worked with would later tell me about the day Mother found out about my hysterectomy. She would walk right out of the church, fall to her knees in the parking lot, pull at her hair while screaming, "HOW COULD SHE DO THIS TO ME?!". I will never understand that story. Logic has no place when dealing with Mother.

After surgery, I was told recovery time would be six to eight weeks. The doctor had cut through my stomach muscles, so I was unable to use stomach muscles for sitting up. I was like a turtle stuck on my back. Brenna moved in with Greg and me during this time to take care of me while Greg was at work. I always thought I would lose Brenna when I quit drugs, but that wasn't the case. She brought over her gaming system for our sleepless nights. We would stay up all night playing video games when the pain kept me awake. Once again, my friends were there to take care of me when family had failed me.

The surgery fixed my pain level but opened up a whole new set of problems. My hormone level was out of balance. My body was trying to go into menopause, and doctors were trying different hormone treatments to prevent this. I was already emotionally unstable, and now I was even more so due to hormonal imbalance. My daily routine would consist of crying episodes or days where I would refuse to get out of bed. Greg developed a relationship with my boss since he would regularly start calling off work for me. Greg suggested therapy to help me during this difficult time.

During my twenties, I would meet with multiple therapists. I would also cycle through jobs thinking that the job was the problem instead of my inability to deal with others. I had already enrolled in massage therapy school since the commercial was repeatedly on the radio. Again, the borderline inside me was easily influenced. I decided that I wanted a job where customers were silent. Mortician school was an hour's drive away, and the massage school was only a thirty-minute drive. This is how I decided to go to massage therapy school. I had also left the credit union to start working as an animal kennel assistant. With all these changes, therapy seemed logical.

My family doctor was already prescribing me anti-depressants to offset the depression caused by hormonal imbalance. I had yet to be diagnosed as a borderline. Unaware that depression and anxiety were common side effects of being a borderline, I took the medication. I was constantly trying different medications, but none offered me relief. I would learn years later that there is no medication for Borderline Personality Disorder. The recommended treatment for Borderline Personality Disorder is Dialectic Behavioral Therapy (DBT). The family doctor made a referral for me to speak to a basic therapist who did not practice DBT. As a borderline, I would chew through multiple therapists before giving up on therapy in my twenties.

The first therapist I always called my bird therapist. She had an unusual amount of bird statues and pictures in her office. It was unsettling to have their dead eyes on me, watching me confess my inner thoughts and feelings. I started with her discussing my issues with hormonal imbalance. She inevitably asked about my family history. Considering I grew up in a house filled with secrets and lies, I couldn't wait to spill my guts about everything that had gone on. Being surrounded by lies makes you more prone to living a life of truth.

Gaslighting always makes you doubt yourself and how you truly remember events. Was I the crazy one in the family? Did I come from a loving family and I was just the ungrateful child? Luckily, I was about to find out. I truly wanted to know if the problem was me, if another child could have gotten along with my family. I still had the letters my mother had sent to me before we stopped talking. I presented them to the therapist, so she had both sides of the story.

Before reading the letters, my therapist stated her goal of helping me maintain a relationship with my family. She said that she would help me be around them while helping me achieve boundaries. The therapist said I could learn to not be affected by them while still maintaining relationships. Then she read Mother's letters.

After reading the letters, her whole plan of action changed. The therapist stated that she couldn't in good conscience recommend that I have any sort of relationship with my family. She commented that no loving mother would have written the letters that I was sent. Mother was deemed a parental failure and a cruel person by a professional therapist. Toxicity was the term used to describe my family.

The human brain cannot understand the difference between feeling the pain of when the assault occurred and remembering the assault. Every time I was placed around those that tried to silence me or assault me, it was like getting attacked all over again. The same synapses and neurons were firing, triggering physiological reactions. This meant every time I had to play "family," my brain would relive the abuse, further damaging me as an adult. This was explained to me by the therapist. It was recommended that I never speak to any of them ever again.

Every day after therapy, I would sit in my car and

cry. Greg would wait for me after the session to hold me. This would be the time I would learn that being sexually assaulted was not my fault. A child is not responsible or accountable for the actions of an adult. It seems like it should be common knowledge. However, in the mind of a trauma victim, it is a concept that is difficult to grasp. You always hold yourself accountable and keep part of the blame on yourself. This was when I was to let go of that blame. Rage was to replace the previous guilt I had felt.

With all therapists, I would inevitably hit a wall. They all seemed wired with the same horrified attitude toward my past. I would always get a lot of "Oh my, that's terrible," or "Dear god, that's horrible!" Yes, hence why I'm in therapy. It just seemed like I was causing therapists to go into therapy. They seemed unable to cope with the nightmares they got from listening to stories of my life.

The second therapist wasn't as fascinated by me as she was fearful. I guess my internal thought processes were alarming to her. She asked to meet with Greg. She made a comment to Greg about her shock at the fact he wasn't scared of me. The revealed fear was comical to me. It wasn't that long until I was counseling that therapist. I was poised to have her confront the cousin that had molested her at Thanksgiving. We were also just starting to get to the root of her daughter's bulimia. Greg canceled that therapist for me. He stated he wasn't going to pay for me to counsel a therapist. I viewed it as an interesting hobby.

Hobbies were the solution offered by my third therapist. She casually threw out the Borderline Personality Disorder diagnosis but never really expanded on it. She recommended Dialectic Behavioral Therapy, but there was no local therapist currently trained in DBT. Her solution to solving the emptiness I felt inside was developing hobbies. I was to give up my need for suicide, my void and lost feeling inside, and find inner peace over some crafty hobby. I had my doubts that something like stamp-collecting was going to solve my life.

Greg took me to Michael's craft store in search of a life-changing hobby. In true borderline extreme fashion, I completed all the hobbies that Michael's had to offer. Woodworking, soap-making, stained glass, cake decorating, whatever was available I completed. It still didn't solve the problem of existing in a normal life after coming from a high-velocity dysfunctional life. Somehow making soap just wasn't as thrilling as racing police cars. Greg tried to find some hobby to entertain me so that he wasn't the only thing in my life. He grew tired of me eternally bothering him for a never-ending supply of attention. The therapist finally told me, "You are as good as you are ever going to be." She had given up. It was becoming common for therapists to quit on me.

I was fired from the vet's office due to my inability to get along with coworkers. I graduated from massage therapy school and got a job in a salon. After a screaming match with the owner, I charged out and was again in between jobs. Greg had returned keys to multiple banks and credit unions for jobs that I refused to go back to. I had quit a video store job by putting my uniform shirt with a nametag in through the night drop box. Sometimes I would walk off jobs just because I just felt like it. I would just decide that I no longer wanted to be there and would leave. I kept thinking it was all about finding the right job. It never occurred to me that the jobs weren't the problem.

Sometimes people try to say that the cycle of jobs is normal and not a borderline thing. However, the extreme reasons behind the cycle is what makes the borderline. I quit one credit union after a failed suicide attempt in the bathroom. The ceiling structure wouldn't support my weight in the noose, and it gave way. Instead of walking back into work from break, I opted for suicide. I just didn't want to work that day, so death seemed like a logical way to not go back to work. Most would look for another job. I was picking myself up off a linoleum bathroom floor to walk back out like nothing was wrong. It would be another job that I would just randomly stop showing up for.

Community college offered a culinary program, so I decided to finally enroll in culinary school. Maybe this would be the way to happiness. I accepted a job at a restaurant to work as a line cook. My chefs would laugh at how my culinary school instructor's background was a supermarket meat cutter. All the chefs at my job had trained in Europe and bypassed culinary school. This was taken into consideration the day I dropped out of school. The moment I got an English teacher that couldn't speak English, I walked out. How was someone who couldn't read English going to grade my papers correctly? My business teacher informed the class he would be late every day due to construction. For some reason, he chose to be late every day instead of just leaving earlier. This was the caliber of teachers that were available. Community college was a bust.

This was the point where Greg gave up on whether I worked or not. He was doing well enough in his career that it didn't matter if I worked or not. I think also my income wasn't worth the hassle of him having to quit jobs for me or call off work for me. He had grown tired of physically dragging me out of bed just to watch me fall to the floor. I would later walk out of the restaurant. I got tired of having talks with chefs about how I had threatened to put coworkers in the trash compactor. My defense that they were flirting with staff, making girls uncomfortable, apparently didn't justify the action.

I explained to the line cooks that I no longer wanted to be there and was thinking of quitting. They all laughed and joked about how they should all walk out. Then they handed me a container of tomatoes and said I should go cut tomatoes before walking out. I chopped the tomatoes, placed the container back on the line, and then walked out of the restaurant. I wonder how long after I left before they realized that I was never joking. It wouldn't be the last job that I would randomly walk out on.

Does a lack of a job make it easier to function as a borderline? I guess it depends on the circumstances. From the outside looking in, I was living the perfect life. I was with a model husband who financially supported me while indulging me in shopping trips to Tiffany & Co. I had gone from homeless to economically secure. This functional life should have been the dream. I now spent most of my time excessively shopping and sleeping the days away in my depression-motivated sleep. Most nights, I would drink a whole bottle of wine and pass out on my backyard deck. This was my marriage.

I have lived on both ends of the financial spectrum. I have been homeless, and I have been wealthy. I have dined at restaurants with my own personal waiter. I have shopped for diamond dog tags from Tiffany & Co. Museum openings, art exhibits, opera guilds, I was in all the right circles. Thank goodness movies like *Pretty Woman* covered table manners. I was able to throw on elaborate ball gowns and not miss a beat with my etiquette learned from TV. It is true what they say: money cannot buy you happiness. One day while shopping, it occurred to me that I had run out of things to buy. Is this why rich people are constantly redoing things they already own? It was at this moment that I decided I wanted a divorce.

Saint Greg was a nickname that was dubbed by friends. The saint part was the most accurate part. Without Greg, I would have never gotten the surgeries that saved my life. Greg stood by me during all the pain, the mood swings, the family drama, and my general everyday uncertainty. He started me on the road to therapy, and it was because of him that I received my diagnosis. The support and love that he offered me was something that I wasn't able to receive. Just as we started as friends, that's how things ended. As friends, we drove to divorce court together and went out to breakfast afterward. Any household item that we both wanted, we flipped a coin over. The lawyer informed Greg that I could have taken him for alimony and made him sell the house so I could have half the proceeds. I opted just to leave with my personal belongings. I explained to Greg that since he bought his first house with his inheritance money, it didn't seem right that I take part of that. I did ask if I could maintain a relationship with his mom. She was the closest to a mother figure that I had ever known. He stated that she had always wanted a daughter, so he was okay with that.

No one would ever understand how I walked away from this seemingly perfect marriage situation. I would explain that I was lonely in a marriage. My brother would tell me, "You are lonely now. At least with Greg, you were lonely with money. Leaving him was the worst decision of your life." People have a hard time understanding that it's more challenging to be alone in a relationship than alone by yourself. I was destined to always feel lonely. It wasn't possible to give me the amount of love that I needed to satiate the starvation I had felt my whole life. All I knew was that Greg was a good person, and I never reconciled the idea of deserving to be with a truly kind soul. I still felt too tainted with evil and unhappiness for anyone in this world.

I was now cycling through jobs in the downtown area. I would bounce around various call center jobs. It made sense to rent a house in the busy downtown area. Greg got me a washer and dryer unit for my new place along with a renter's insurance policy. He wanted to make sure I was set up okay. On some snowy days, he would swing by my house in the morning and clean the snow off my car. Forever the saint.

Living by myself was learning about who I was as a person. I had spent so long trying to fit into different molds. People that have endured trauma are experts at being chameleons. Blending in makes it easier to be overlooked for a person's rage or abuse. I was so busy trying to blend in that I never had time to stop and figure out who I was as a person. All I knew was that as a person, I felt dead inside. I was in a brand-new place once again rebuilding my life.

I spent four hours in the shower curtain aisle at a store. I didn't even know what shower curtain design my personal style was. I stood there openly crying in the aisle, refusing to leave until I selected one. All these different personalities and I had to find out what shower curtain would appease all of them. This was my level of brokenness. I struggled to pick out a shower curtain. To this day, I still have the decorated shower curtain hook that I chose. It was a whimsical pattern with pink sparkles. It was the first of many decisions, and all of them would be this difficult.

After a year of renting the house, I decided to buy my own home. I had gotten two dogs named Ginger and Cherry. They were both German Shepherd mixes. I wanted to give them a beautiful backyard to run in. I informed my realtor that I was buying a house for my dogs. She thought I was kidding until she learned I was only interested in viewing the back yard first. Even though they were inside dogs, I still wanted a lovely outdoor play area for them. If it wasn't acceptable, then I would pass on seeing the remainder of the home, no matter how nice it was. Eventually, she got on board and found me a perfect house with a beautiful fenced-in yard.

When I was a child, my parents got me a beagle dog. They kept the beagle, Muffins, in the laundry room. My father cut a hole in the door and made a window so the dog could look out. If you wanted to see the dog, you would look at it through this little window. Mother's bichon poodle dog got free run of the house while my dog was trapped in the laundry room. I was determined to give my current dogs a better life.

I made a logical choice in my home purchase but

should have considered the emotional side of it. I looked around many cities trying to decide where to buy. The difference in taxes from city to city was factored into this decision. In the end, I chose a house that was seven streets over from my parents' house, my original home. I was able to live there for two years before they knew. I thought I would only be there temporarily before selling the house and moving again. Sadly, this is when the national mortgage crisis happened, and my home value plummeted. I was now in a more permanent living situation.

I was twenty-nine years old when I bought my first house. The day I moved in, I dropped to the floor and lay down in the middle of the empty room. Home. It was my first real home. It was also the first time that I had officially unpacked all my personal belongings. I had gotten used to keeping certain things in boxes, considering how much I moved around when I was homeless. I was twenty-nine and had never felt safe or stable enough to unpack my belongings until now. My furnishings were still minimal, but I loved how much open space that gave me. At that moment, I was happy.

Even after working with multiple therapists, I could not allow myself to stay happy. Happiness is an unsettling feeling to those that aren't used to feeling it. Instead of waiting, I pulled the rug out from underneath my own self. I started dating a guy who was the opposite of Greg. The saintly character was nowhere to be found with this gentleman caller named Drew.

My relationship with Drew was a common borderline relationship. My manic states were more common in dysfunctional relationships. At one point, I went out and purchased eight cats in one day. The house had kittens everywhere, which was entertaining until I came down from mania. Then I had the chore of rehoming eight cats. In my manic state, I had forgotten that I was allergic to cats.

It was a constant push-pull of me ending and restarting my relationship with Drew. I would push buttons so hard that Drew would physically fight me. He would choke me out while dragging me down the hallway. This relationship was toxic. During one argument, in anger, he pointed out that I had no family. I marched right out the front door to my mother's house. It was at this point that I brought her back into my life. Just for sport to fight with Drew, I unleashed Mother. Mother had no issues with tearing apart Drew and his life choices. One would think that she was standing up for her daughter, but this wasn't the case. She honestly just loved a good fight. It was like owning a rabid dog. You turn the dog loose on your enemy and hope that the focus stays on them instead of turning on you. But that dog would always turn. In my need to hurt Drew, I didn't think far enough ahead in my choice to bring her back around.

I ended up marrying Drew and divorced him five months later. There was no post-divorce breakfast like there was for Greg and me. I informed him at the courthouse that he was to go before the judge and agree to my terms. If he tried to refuse me, I told him that I would leave him at the courthouse and people would show up and break his legs. Not wanting to crawl home from court, he agreed to the divorce.

Relationships with men came and went as often as I changed career fields. I had been working in call centers but was now on short-term disability from work. My recent therapist approved my paperwork since she never wanted me around people at all. Based on my life story, she stated she was just happy I didn't "end up in a clocktower." My response was, "I'm still young and have time."

My most recent boss had tried to get me fired for attendance, but I had been keeping copies of every email she sent regarding her leaving work early. She liked to spend time with her grandson. When she tried to get me in trouble, I presented my folder of all her time off to her boss. I got to keep my job, and she had to start copying her boss on all emails. I learned over time how to keep my jobs. Subtle blackmailing was fine with me.

After my short-term disability ran out, I worked in the jewelry field. I managed the diamond inventory but had to leave that job because I couldn't get along with yet another manager. With a background in diamonds and money, I ended up working for an armored car service in one of their cash houses. Now I had a job with a gun.

Cash houses are places where banks store their

money. It was nothing to have to balance two million dollars in cash a day. The irony was not lost on the fact that the hustler was now in charge of large cash quantities. Even more comical was when local police tried to recruit me from the work-enforced gun school. I was called a natural shooter. Being able to shoot right- or left-handed, one-handed, in the dark, in flashing lights: it's a skill I learned I had. When they first talked to me about being a paid shooter, I thought, "Finally! A job as an assassin!" When I learned it was for their SWAT team, I passed. I still viewed myself more as a villain than in the role of a hero. Later, I would walk out of that job after tossing my gun in some random work locker.

Retail, insurance, banking, culinary, massage therapy, jewelry, private security: my jobs were all over with no pattern. The only pattern was me not keeping one long term. Mother would say I was a "jack of all trades." I would say that I was so damaged with broken people skills that I was set up to fail at life. No career path could be had. The jobs were not the problem. Working as a person with Borderline Personality Disorder was indeed a problem for me. As much of a mess as the job situation was, at least my bills were getting paid. I had at least twenty resumes. I could shift from one job field to the next. Stories were fictionalized to explain gaps in employment and reasons for the change in a career field. I have easily had over a hundred jobs in my lifetime. This chaotic mess was still more organized than my love life.

After my experience with Drew, my interest in dating was minimal. I was never an avid dater to begin with. My friends would tell me that I must get out there because Mr. Right won't just knock at your door. Their hands went up in the air when neighbors started ringing my doorbell to ask me out. It was so convenient. I didn't even need to leave my house to find people to date. The people I met dating just made me feel like I had an invisible bat signal to lure all the crazies in.

I would date someone who informed me he was taking himself off antipsychotic medication. I was unaware he was even on medication. He felt this was the only way to get along with his other personality named Machine. According to him, Machine had homicidal tendencies. At this point, he also started making music with his cat. I slowly stepped away. Far be it for me to come between him and the future career of Cat Benatar.

I would meet another who would want me to go with him to cemeteries to dig up bones, so he would have authentic skull décor for his house. He just needed me to go on a late-night hike with him into the woods with a shovel. I wasn't sure I would have come back from that hike. Politely I declined and suggested seeing other people. Over time, I developed a top five list of the craziest people I had ever dated.

You had to be more than a garden-variety stalker to make my top five. The person in the number one spot resulted in me talking to the government about his impending revolution. The surprise was on me when I showed up, and he was building explosives to "change the world." I couldn't even change myself, and here he was trying to change the whole damn world. Ironically, ATF approved for him to have silencers on all his firearms. This approval happened after his eviction from a school for threatening to shoot it up. He had shot and wounded a friend in a bar fight just to be approved later for a conceal carry gun permit. As pro-gun as I am, I do agree there has to be more of a tighter screening process. He had guns, I had guns. It seemed like all the crazy people were running around with guns.

If I didn't have Post Traumatic Stress Disorder before, dating ensured that I had it now. It was now common practice to run people's names through the criminal database before accepting a date. Dating seemed lethal, and the jobs were disappointing. By this point, I chose to fall into a bottle and drink my life away. When starting to frequent local bars, I reconnected with a high school friend named David.

David was perfect for me. He was an ideal partner to go out with since he came with zero romantic complications. David was gay and one of the few people in this life that accepted me just the way I was. David knew me during my street racer days and still never judged me. He would drag me along to join him rollerblading. Being against a healthy lifestyle, I was only there for the promise of ice cream after this excursion. He would laugh at the fact that I would smoke while rollerblading.

We were quite the pair. His laid-back, accepting attitude made it easy for him to get along with people. We were opposites in that respect since I hated interacting with anyone. I always admired his people skills and how people just naturally loved him. Many were unaware that this loving-life attitude came from his being terminally diagnosed, with HIV. He was just enjoying the ride till the end. I fell right in step next to him. He would enjoy life, while I was always awaiting death.

My time with David would accelerate my level of drinking alcohol. I needed an ungodly amount of alcohol just to bring me down and level me out, to make me feel normal. David was the only one who could keep up and drink on my level. We would watch everyone pass out at parties and then we would try to make it to the bar for last call. Everyone was considered a lightweight drinker to us. I had switched from drugs to drinking to endure life. After closing out the bar, we would stay up all night cooking gourmet feasts to soak up the alcohol. Our nights cooking together are some of my favorite memories.

During this time, I also started learning how to eat fire. The joy of YouTube videos! My newest hobby was fire spinning. I watched some videos, ordered a fire staff—among other props—and jumped right in. Fire was to be my new toy. I would occasionally get gigs performing. David was beyond proud. He would take his laptop into bars to show his coworkers and friends my performances. He was the most supportive person that I had in my life. When I was recruited to audition for the circus, David would say, "Well, it was only a matter of time before you ran away with the circus."

I trained on the trapeze with the circus but never developed it into a job. It always required a severe amount of trust to fall and be caught by the hands of strangers. Trust was not something that I was great at. Others would view these hobbies as extreme, but to me, they provided a calmness. I felt Zen-like trance come over me as I was surrounded by fire. David would ask, "How can you perform while people are taking pictures with so many camera flashes?" I would reply, "People were taking my picture?" Everything fell away when I spun fire. Later in life, I would learn that these hobbies were my subconscious trying to shock my system awake to feel something, to feel anything. Still, falling through the sky catching a trapeze bar, I felt nothing.

While David was cheering me on, Mother reverted back to a kid sister figure. She would continuously be angry that I wouldn't teach her fire or perform with her. Her ideas of a mother daughter combo pair sounded like the stuff of nightmares. Instead of feeling pride, all she ever felt was envy. The longing for all eyes to be on her was the exact opposite reason I spun fire. I was spinning to obtain the feeling of falling and fading away.

My love of fire would spill over into the artists'

community. The talent of these young kids is inspiring. They needed a safe space to develop their craft. I would work with a partner to establish a fire center for youth to learn and practice. Fire performers are usually on the younger side, so most live in apartments. It's difficult to practice hula-hooping a fire hoop in a one-bedroom without taking out your television. Later I would pass on the center to my partner and move on to other things.

Throughout the whole fire center process, mother would scream about how the community center shouldn't be built. She would rant about how I was to be sued, or my partner would betray me. My partner and I would agree on things based on a handshake. Having a partnership purely based on trust was something she could never understand. She trusted no one. Her childish tantrum failed to derail this project. The kids ended up with their fire center.

Recovery

✳

Was I alive? Maybe I was just an empty shell walking through life imitating life. The constant movement of jumping in and out of different social circles was exhausting. It was a constant race pushing myself forward but with no destination. The various personalities of each scene were struggling to keep up the façade of normalcy. I was engaging with life and building relationships, but it all felt false. It was as if I was playing pretend at life since I still felt empty and hollow inside. Was my life just to be a constant cycling of jobs and hobbies with no inner peace?

The excessive drinking encouraged a party life that helped me run at max speed. Or at least I thought my drinking had me maxed out. I had no idea how much more I could be ramped up in the drinking lifestyle until I took a job as a server. The most basic of jobs had the most profound impact on my life.

David would indirectly introduce me to the third guy I would become engaged to. We would never make it down the aisle, due to his cheating. Between cycling jobs and failing at another relationship, I decided to go back to school. I thought if I had a career to throw myself into, then I would no longer have time to waste on dating people. Dating seemed so pointless since it always ended in disappointment. I never felt worthy of love.

After scanning the college curriculum, I enrolled as a surgical technician student. Mother would tell people I was going to school to be a doctor. My choices were still below her standards. She always loved any job I had that would give her a discount on things. By the time I left the jewelry store, she probably owned half their inventory. Naturally, I applied for a server job at Olive Garden. It was the one restaurant that Mother hated eating at, so it was a safe choice.

The head manager told me he liked me within two minutes of talking to him. I told him how I was in a two-year college program, and he could have me as an employee for two years. He agreed, and we shook on it. *Bueno Festa!* I was now a member of the Olive Garden family. Here I was, a server in my thirties being trained by servers in their twenties. I made sure my work shirts were ironed and starched. My shirts had that precise, crisp line down the sleeve. I was armed with a Tide bleach pen in my apron for potential pasta spills. My apron pocket also contained an assortment of colorful pens. I even ironed my necktie, committed to doing the best possible job. I went from negotiating loans for a client's private jet to learning how to make all the teas to drink at Olive Garden.

Before every shift, I would look at myself in the mirror. I would give myself a pep talk on how I can do this. I am a successful person that will learn to carry trays of drinks. I will learn to carry trays of food without throwing them everywhere. Then one day, it happened. I spilled a tray of sticky sweet raspberry lemonade beverages all over customers at a table. Of course, this happened in front of the head manager that hired me. I felt sick to my gut. I couldn't do a basic thing and knew that I was going to be fired. I felt like a failure. The kind of failure that parents hate. The kind of failure that can't keep a relationship. The kind of failure that people cheat on. The kind of failure that cannot manage a simple task of carrying drinks from point A to point B. My borderline brain was already escalating the situation in my mind. I considered walking out at that moment. The manager called me over and asked if this was the first tray I had spilled. I apologized and stated it was. A slow smile appeared over his face. He raised his hand, offering me a high five. "Welcome to the industry!" he stated. With those words, I could breathe again. Servers were approaching me on smoke breaks, offering me tips on carrying trays. One server kept telling me in the alley... "You got this! It's all in your head!". Then I realized, I was becoming an Olive Garden server.

School had started and so had my two-year countdown. Each day was a struggle to get out of bed due to my depression and anxiety. I would look around my job and wonder what did I have in common with any of these kids? They were just starting out in life. They were just starting down the education path toward a new future. Then I realized what we did have in common. We were coworkers. Coworkers working toward a better future for ourselves. Coworkers that supported each other and shared crazy customer stories to pass the time and make for laughter during the workday. This was when I realized that I needed to embrace my new life.

Most server shifts are about four hours long. These short shifts are ideal for people that are dealing with depression or anxiety issues. It is easier to get out of bed knowing you only work four hours. On days where you can't even manage four hours, you can post your shift, and a server will pick it up for you. This significantly reduced my attendance problems. Some servers are lifers in this field due to the daily struggle of depression and anxiety. Another reason customers should be kind to those who refill your water. People never know the demons a person is dealing with.

It's a fast-paced, chaos-filled environment that randomly comes to a dead halt when the dinner rush is over, and you are sent home. Of course, you are wound up and still have energy to burn off before you can wind down. This is what creates the other side of the server environment. The environment of burning off steam. House parties after work are a standard in the server industry. It's a time to vent about your day, vent about management, and bond with your team by consuming mass quantities of alcohol. Suddenly, I was in a work environment where I could thrive, and my drinking was viewed as normal.

Server drinking adventures would even take place in the form of road trips. I would travel to an out-of-state comic con to meet David Tennant from *Doctor Who* with another server. I was that crazy fan that made him buckeye candy. We would create cosplay costumes and run around the comic con event all weekend. After we agreed to try comic con speed dating, she went out on a date with one of her matches. I opted to throw away my list of matches and drink it up at the afterparty event.

Another server had me visit her in another state to support her during her divorce. With a suitcase filled with Pedialyte and Zofran, we would drink all weekend for fourteen hours straight at a time. We would crash hotel pools while bar-hopping. After hitting multiple bars, we entered a sword shop and walked out armed with katana swords. In *Kill Bill* fashion, we jumped on the back of random strangers' motorcycles and raced through a tourist town drunk, katanas strapped on our back. Monday, we were back to smiling at guests while asking if they wanted refills.

My reputation for drinking led to my house becoming a server destination for after-work parties. Drinks would pour, and servers would light up my fire toys to spin off their excess energy. I built a fire pit for bonfires, replaced my dinette with a stripper pole in my kitchen, and always had vodka in stock. For New Year's, we built a balloon-drop system in my living room complete with confetti cannons. During a pirate-themed party, nearby neighbors randomly jumped over the backyard fence to join in the festivities. The parties were getting so big and extreme that there were now crashers. The energy level was equal to the manic borderline thoughts racing through my head.

This was the first job where I connected with people. Over time, my house shifted from being a party destination to a server sanctuary. I would console those who would show up crying over school stress and lost loves. There would be discussions about planned moves or contemplated career changes. My house transitioned to a caring, safe environment for those in need. I would put blankets over those that had passed out crying from arguing with their parents. I didn't realize it at the time, but I had created a safe place for those who struggled with life. It was the shelter I wish I had found when I was struggling. Years later, I would stay in touch with those who had moved on in life. On one vacation trip, a friend's fiancée would tell me, "The only happy stories James has about Ohio involves times at your house." Those words would forever ring in my ears.

I went to singing contests to support my coworkers as they dealt with stage fright. I practiced lines with coworkers in the alley to help them prepare for an upcoming acting audition. I would watch these kids with their study cards in the drink stations. In between tables, they would study for their upcoming exams. I have quizzed so many servers on anything from nursing exams to computer certifications. We had one girl who needed to assemble and train a full choir for her master's program. She had just moved to the area and barely knew anyone. Yes, we had an Olive Garden choir. The managers even scheduled around everyone's choir practices. All these events would have an audience packed with servers. They always made sure there was a cheering section to support their own.

School support wasn't the only love these servers showed each other. One server had her purse stolen during Christmas time. I watched all the servers open their wallets and kick in toward her family Christmas. If someone had car problems, they always found rides with coworkers. We grieved together when dealing with a server who opted to take his own life. People would cry in the back of the store before wiping tears away to go smile for customers. When servers are sick or hospitalized, they can't work. This means they don't make any money. The servers raise money for their own. I drove one server to the hospital. I held the hand of a scared girl about to undergo an emergency appendectomy. I went through her phone to call her mom to notify her that her daughter was in the hospital and she was needed. In her face, I saw my younger face holding the same fear that I had before my surgery.

The single moms partnered up to create their own daycare system. They would alternate babysitting each other's kids to ensure people could pick up the shifts they needed. The mom squad would set up play dates for their kids. These kids were being raised in an Olive Garden. Mandatory employee meetings would consist of servers and sometimes their kids too. They would host baby showers and wedding showers. I have even seen coworkers fall in love. We would go to their weddings. A few years later, we would be visiting them in the hospital to welcome the birth of their first child. Pictures of these events would be taken by an aspiring photographer who worked at our Olive Garden. The support and love they showed each other was unlike anything I had ever known.

Years in the finance world, and I never received that kind of support. That world was filled with backstabbing office politics. People who smiled in your face while trying to steal your accounts. I had never known people who were genuinely supportive of their teammates until this job. The last time I had seen this level of support was during my short exposure to the world of exotic dancers. Why are the jobs that are viewed by society as the worst, filled by the best people?

The personal struggles I witnessed help put my life in perspective. Yes, my brain is wired differently. Yes, I struggle with people due to having Borderline Personality Disorder. But I watched as servers struggled with their sexuality. I had server friends who were dealing with being transgender. They reminded me of my *Rocky Horror* friends that got lost along the way. I learned of the battles of health care for obtaining hormone treatment and the expenses of name changing. I learned about the fear they faced in everyday life. The fear of family rejecting them. The fear of being bullied or harassed. The fear of never finding love. These were fears that we shared. The managers had no issues changing their names and supporting this change. Acceptance was something that never ran short at Olive Garden.

Some servers were arrested based on alcohol and drug issues. Everyone came together in support. They did not lose their job. Instead, they gained a network of people that cared. Servers that had earned their sobriety chips reached out to help those in need. They had been down that road and knew exactly what those who were struggling needed. The money was not the main reason people chose to work there. Other restaurants had higher checks, resulting in larger tips. These people were here because they truly loved the environment. This is the family that the Olive Garden commercials spoke of.

I worked for Olive Garden for five years. It was the longest I ever held the same job. It was the first time I felt connected to others. I felt inspired by their hopes and dreams. I saw my own pain in their struggles. Their stories of pain and triumphs moved my soul. I wasn't finding that feeling at the hospital. I decided to drop out of school with two weeks till graduation. I chose to spend my last financial aid check on a PlayStation 4 instead of completing my degree. I held a 4.0 grade point average and threw it away. When I did my clinical rotation in the operating room, I learned the job wasn't for me. I never planned on leaving Olive Garden. Sadly, a new manager showed up, and that was when I left. Once again, I just couldn't get along with a manager. This time it was because I couldn't stand to see how difficult she was making life for the servers. It broke my heart.

I can honestly say Olive Garden saved me. More accurately, the people I met while working there saved me. It was through these connections that I was able to build healthy friendships and find the love of my life. I was to receive a marriage proposal prompted by giving someone an Olive Garden breadstick. But before finding him, I found her. I had Ellen move in with me as a roommate.

I met Ellen while working at Olive Garden. We became friends while having drinks on a ski trip with a group of coworkers. Ellen had a dark sense of humor that I adored. After that weekend, we started to spend time together regularly. She was struggling to get along with her parents, so I offered her a place to stay. I thought having a roommate might keep me from getting so caught up with my negative thoughts. When I have too much quiet time, the voices in my head get super loud. Quiet time spins me out of control and makes me ponder suicide. The previous party house I had lived in supplied me with roommates. This was a different situation. It was almost as if I had turned back time and was doing things the right way. I had a healthy roommate situation. No dealing, no hiding people from the police, no hiding cars that had been used in crimes, just normal day-to-day living. We both just worked as servers and paid bills.

The time Ellen lived with me meant the world to me. I enjoyed our late-night talks and bonding over binge-watching cooking shows. Our days off together involved brunches, skiing, or just playing video games in our pajamas. She was also great at helping me take care of the dogs. She even bought a pet bed for her bedroom floor in case one of the dogs wanted to visit her in her room. Despite all the partying and drinking, my home environment felt safe.

Another benefit of having Ellen live with me was that it kept Mother away. She never liked coming around if there were others around to witness her craziness. Ellen only met my mother twice in her lifetime. She stated that within five minutes of meeting Mother, she "wanted to crawl into a bottle and die." It sounded like a typical response since that's how Mother always made me feel.

Ellen struggled with her own mental health issues,

so she was very understanding of mine. She had met mother, and based on the interaction, Ellen stated she now knew why I was so unbalanced. I would talk to Ellen about us moving to another state. Every day was a different state. I would show her pictures of the apartments that I found, and she would always say how great it was. But with all the different fractured parts of yourself, when you are constantly in flux, how do you make a choice? Ellen was aware of this and knew that a move wouldn't happen, but she still indulged my talks.

I would try and make myself feel more permanent in my home environment. I painted a black Jolly Roger flag covering a whole wall in my house. I thought if I painted a wall black while knowing it's the hardest color to cover, I would finally accept that this was my permanent residence. Still, it never felt permanent, even when I painted a Union Jack flag on the other wall. It also never felt permanent when I painted my bedroom orange with black outlined figures from the movie *A Clockwork Orange*. I still wanted to push forward with no known destination, and nothing could make me accept the calmness of staying still. The paint was spilling out the way a dam releases water to reduce pressure. But I was running out of walls to paint.

It was during this time that my dog Cherry suffered a stroke. Her legs were not working, and she was unable to walk. Ellen ramped up her work hours to cover my half of the bills. She told me to "stay home and take care of our girl." In our house the dogs were family. Cherry had outlasted two husbands and a fiancé. She was more reliable for support and love than any human. She had been in my life for twelve years, which is longer than any person.

I would lift this fifty-pound dog up in a harness with one arm. This freed up my other hand to move each of her legs to simulate walking. I wanted to make sure she wouldn't develop blood clots while recovering. An Olive Garden server who was also a nursing student would stop by to take Cherry's vitals. Servers would use their employee meals to order a steak to send to my house for Cherry. I would change Cherry's diapers and hold her head up so she could eat and drink. I wanted to give her scrambled brain time to recover from her seizure.

The vet advised Cherry to be put down if she didn't walk by that Thursday. On Thursday, she got up and walked on her own. Ellen and I hugged and cried tears of happiness. Mother happened to be over when this event occurred. She had been campaigning for me to put Cherry down. The first words out of her mouth were, "Well, sometimes they get better before they get worse." Ellen told me later that she has never wanted to punch someone in the mouth as much as my mother. It was then that Ellen stated she never wanted to be around my mother again. I shared the same feeling. Cherry passed away four years later at the age of sixteen.

My involvement with Mother was minimal at this time. My brother had been released from prison with his brand-new swastika tattoo. Mother was nice enough to present him with a bill on his release from prison. She had been keeping track of the mileage for all her visits to the prison, the phone calls, the money placed on his books and various other things. The whole time he was in there, he thought she was being supportive. Getting a bill for supportive services was not what he was expecting.

I grew tired of hearing about my brother from mother. I explained that hearing about him made me uncomfortable, but she didn't care. All she wanted to talk about was how great he was doing in his new life. He met a girl online who had four kids of her own. He moved to Australia and married her. They had two more kids, making for six kids in total. I'm still struggling with everyday functioning, but he was doing great. Not really the conversation I wanted to hear. Every time she brought him up, all it did was remind me of being assaulted and how there was no punishment for any of my abusers. They all went on with their happy lives after destroying any hope I had to be a functioning adult. There was no justice.

Mother had found the perfect sad story to spin for drama. She would now cry to anyone who would listen about the struggles of her grandkids being so far away. It was if she now liked children. I'm not sure where that side of her was when I was growing up. She never looked at those kids and realized that they were the same innocent age I was when I was abused. It leads me to believe that once again, it was all for show. She would now Skype with the kids and send boxes of presents. The Skype time also allowed her to tell him how he should raise his kids and deal with his wife. Suddenly, she was the expert on parenting, and my brother was actually listening to her.

My family had become so involved with celebrating a new life. I couldn't fathom why someone would want to pass on our genes. Why would anyone celebrate being born into this family? Our family was filled with child molesters, mental health problems, and bad genes. The responsible, educated choice would be to adopt instead of passing that on to children. This celebration of life was also difficult to understand when I was currently surrounded by death. David's health was declining. My surrogate family was once again slipping through my fingers.

My past lifestyle had trained me to view friends as temporary. So many were lost to prison and drugs. Losing David shattered a part of my soul. He was my match in life. I felt spun out without a partner. His decline was rapid as he ended up in hospice care. People poured in to say their goodbyes as I kept my distance. How could I say goodbye? After being there for a few days, I finally took my turn to talk to him. Even on life support, he could hear me. I just knew it. It wasn't till I said my goodbye that he departed this earth. I believe he was waiting to hear from me before leaving. I'm thankful for every day he clung to life to give me time to build up the strength to say goodbye. But I'm more grateful for having known him.

David had lived with his grandmother. Since his parents lacked child-raising skills, she was the one who raised him. Everyone always saw the party side of him. The side I saw was the part that regularly played *Jeopardy* with his grandmother. Because of my love for him, I would routinely check on her to make sure she was doing okay. Every time I left her house, my fake smile would fall away and be replaced with tears. Visiting that house was always painful, knowing he wasn't there. But in life, sometimes taking care of others is difficult.

Mother never checked on me after the loss of David. She still viewed HIV as a gay disease. Her attitude was, "Well, that's what comes with being gay." Ellen escorted me to the funeral. She made us large travel mugs of Irish coffee to get us through. Plus, I think David would have approved of us drinking in his honor, even though his drink was cherry vodka with Sprite. My world dimmed after his loss. It would never be as bright without him.

David careened through this life at lightning speed. I was grateful that toward the end of his time, he got to meet Darrin. Darrin was to be my future husband, unbeknownst to me at the time. It was if the universe understood that one partner was going to be leaving me; therefore, it introduced to me another. I would meet Darrin randomly after one of my shifts at Olive Garden.

An Olive Garden breadstick would bring us together.

After my nightly work shift, I would go through a drive-thru to pick up a pack of cigarettes. A nasty and expensive habit, I admit. I would quit years later and miss it daily. I decided to change which drive-thru I went to since the regular cashier was getting too chatty for my taste. I pulled into the new drive-thru and was greeted by a guy named Darrin.

Darrin would tell me later that he was intimidated by me because I was always leading this exciting life. He would see skis in my car for weekend trips or fire props for gigs. Multiple Olive Garden servers would come through the drive-thru to buy mixers on their way to my house for parties. He mistakenly thought I had a busy social life, but it was just an illusion. The reality was this socializing was just my inner borderline racing through life. He thought I was standoffish because I was antisocial. Being around strangers gives me anxiety. I always want to get in and out of the stores quickly. Having Post Traumatic Stress Disorder makes going out in public a battle. The fear of being attacked was an ongoing issue that I had to overcome daily.

One day while getting my cigarettes, I offered Darrin some Olive Garden food that was my employee meal for the night. It was the first kind, social gesture that I had made to him. He raved about loving their breadsticks and proposed to me. We didn't even know each other's names. Whenever I would stop for cigarettes, it was our running joke of us calling each other fiancé. I knew what it was like to work in shops where you were just surrounded by junk food. You crave real food for snacking. Darrin viewed it as an act of kindness and was touched. He was hooked.

Darrin was thirty-one years old when we met. I was thirty-eight years old and used to dating guys in their twenties. Based on my appearance, most people guessed me to be around thirty-two years old. Somehow the drugs and drinking hadn't aged me. Still, he was considered too old for me to date. Dating younger guys ensured they would keep up with my party lifestyle. They were also viewed as safer candidates since the ability to be serious with them wasn't an option. Darrin was not even on my radar as a potential candidate to date.

One day I came through the drive-thru with a friend that went to high school with Darrin. After that, Darrin was a known, vetted person. No longer was he some random customer service person. This is how Darrin secured an invite to my next house party. He would show up to see people hanging upside down on a stripper pole. Outside there were fire spinners and someone grilling up food for everyone. There was his choice of alcoholic cupcakes or cannabis fudge for desserts. This scene, at times, would scare suitors off, with haste. Most people that show up for a cookout do not expect this type of environment. Darrin jumped right in and made friends. I was both surprised and intrigued.

It wasn't long before Darrin and I started spending all our free time together. He moved in with Ellen and me within a few months. Ellen suggested that since he was at the house most of the time that he should just move in. Almost immediately after that, he wanted to meet my family. Darrin viewed this as a way to express his serious intent of our future together. I saw it as a recipe for disaster. The request was denied.

Darrin learned what my family was like when he escorted me to the hospital for my father's surgery. After Mother's feeding him a lifetime supply of biscuits and gravy, he repeatedly required having arteries cleaned out. This time he was also having a pacemaker put in. Darrin would chat with mother in the surgery waiting room. He got up to take the elevator to the parking garage for a cigarette break. The moment the elevator doors closed, mother turned to me. The first thing she said was, "Is he wearing your T-shirt? Is that why he dates big girls, to wear their clothes?". I opted to not reply and just join Darrin for a smoke break. After informing Darrin what was said, we had sex in the hospital parking garage just as a big fuck you response to the world. Darrin would start to pass on future interactions with my family.

After a few months of Darrin living with me, Ellen moved out. Ellen had been the anchor keeping the borderline in check. Now that she was gone, things shifted from three roommates living together to me being in a serious relationship. This kind of situation is what always leads me to cracking. When Ellen left, Darrin and I started fighting. Despite all the push-pull of our relationship, Darrin still wanted to marry me. He proposed to me on St Patrick's Day when we were out celebrating with our friends. Mother would claim it was not a real proposal because we must have been drunk. She changed her tune when she realized I had an engagement ring, and this was a real thing.

I was to be married for the third time. Our wedding would take place in our living room with a justice of the peace officiating and two of our friends as witnesses. I explicitly stated that no family would be included. I made flower collars for the dogs and put a GoPro on one of them to film it. We called her the viDOGrapher. It was a simple ceremony, and it suited us perfectly. Afterward, we went to dinner with our friends and started our life as a married couple.

Marriage does not fix relationships. Both Darrin and I had been married before and were aware of this. We knew that this would be work, but the arguing was getting worse. Darrin would try to express his side of an argument. I would take this as him trying to make everything about him the way that Mother did. In reality, he was just explaining his side to me so we could find a compromise in the middle. All this did was trigger the borderline rage to come out. The rage that I felt toward mother ignoring my life and making everything about her was projected onto Darrin.

The hate and rage I felt toward my family were

welcomed by Darrin with open arms. The interesting part about Darrin was he had a history of his own personal trauma and abuse. He knew my struggles and the demons I fought with daily. He had also undergone extensive anger management and stress relief courses to get a handle on his own battles. Nothing I did was scaring off Darrin. This included a fight during which I held a gun to Darrin's head, threatening to end his life.

Darrin was not the first person I had ever threatened with a firearm. This was, however, the incident that made me realize something had to change. Here I was again, angry at life and spinning out of control. Mother was back trying to pit me against Darrin's mother for her own personal competition. This time I had recognized her spin-control game and opted out. She would even go as far as stating that Greg's mother agreed with her on things. The hope was that by using Greg's mom as leverage, she could still make me spin. But I knew Greg's mom better than she did. Greg's mother maintained her Facebook friendship with Mother to keep tabs on her for my protection. That lady didn't have a thread of evil in her soul, so I didn't believe what mother was saying.

Mother would eventually be banned from my house. Darrin was the first person to not indulge my mother. He would not play nice to her face and then talk behind her back. He had no problem calling her out for her unacceptable behavior. Suddenly I had a defender, someone to stand up for me when my voice was beaten down. The turning point came during Cherry's final days.

Cherry's health was declining as a sixteen-year-old dog. Mother stopped by to explain that she was having surgery on her eyes. I didn't have time to indulge her by listening to her regarding another operation of vanity. I was busy trying to syringe Pedialyte into Cherry's mouth for her diarrhea. Mother looked at Cherry and said, "Why don't you die and stop being a burden on your mother?" I threw her out and texted Darrin about what happened since he was at work. Darrin was livid.

Darrin messaged Mother forbidding her from coming to the house. He stated that this was his family to protect and love. If she couldn't treat people with kindness and respect, then she had no business coming around. He tore into her for attacking Cherry since he viewed Cherry as his child. If I chose to interact with my mother, then that was my choice. However, it would not be at our home. I was unaware that Darrin messaged Mother, Mother was back at my front door within five minutes.

She was raging about the message Darrin had sent her. I informed her that if she had a problem with Darrin, she should take it up with him. From the very beginning, I always told Darrin that I would back him up over my family. He knew that he never had to hold back or refrain from expressing his feelings toward them. They never had my loyalty. This was the last time

Mother would be at my house. Darrin was the first person in history to go toe to toe with my mother and come out a winner.

Having Darrin support me and stand by me was new to me. Others would always smile at Mother then talk behind her back. This allowed her the feeling that she was in the right, and I was indeed the crazy one. Never being called out for her bad behavior just encouraged the years of her being destructive and abusive. After years of others reinforcing this behavior, it's hard to cling to the fact that you aren't the crazy one. Others' politeness was indirectly harming me more than helping. Now I didn't feel so alone in the world anymore. I had a partner. A partner that would stand up and shame her for her treatment of those she claimed to love. He was to shed his light onto the darkness, banishing it from existence. Darrin became my hero.

Being around Greg's family always made me feel worse about myself. Darrin never pushed me to be around his family. He never pushed me to do anything outside my comfort zone. He was just accepting of any part of myself that I could offer. I never felt good enough for Greg. Was I ready for a lasting marriage with Darrin? Before David died, he met Darrin. He would tell me how great he thought Darrin was and would ask me, "Do you even date nice guys?" It was a valid question. How was I to prevent another failed marriage? Darrin did not deserve a gun put to his head in rage. When he bowed his head in submissiveness stating his inner peace with impending death, it was my wake-up call. I needed help.

Every partner I had previously been involved with wanted me in therapy or on medication. Darrin is the only person that required neither. He accepted me as the broken person I was. It was up to me if I wanted to become a better person or remain as I was. I knew the path if there was no change. This was when I went to search for help for my Borderline Personality Disorder. Darrin deserved better, and I wanted to feel like I deserved Darrin. I wanted to feel like I deserved love.

There is no medication for Borderline Personality Disorder. There is medication for Post Traumatic Stress Disorder, but my BPD symptoms would override that. SSRIs would either make my anxiety and depression worse or the pills would have no effect. Therefore, I couldn't even take medication for that condition. I recently had surgery to remove my gallbladder and was now unable to drink. My excessive drinking had finally killed my gallbladder. Without that buffer, I wasn't comfortable drinking. I knew I was now killing my liver. I was going through life without a crutch. This was a time for panic.

Previous experience had taught me that therapy was pointless since most were ill-equipped to deal with my level of trauma. But what about a therapist that was skilled in Dialectical Behavioral Therapy? I had been told that was the best treatment for borderlines. When I was in my twenties, I searched for a therapist with this skillset. The nearest one was a three-hour drive away from me. That seemed excessive for a weekly treatment. I hadn't searched for one since my twenties. Things had changed since then.

Marsha M. Linehan, Ph.D., ABPP is the creator of treatment for people with Borderline Personality Disorder. The treatment is called Dialectical Behavior Therapy (DBT). She is a skilled psychologist and distinguished author who has won many notable honors and awards. Such credits include the Louis Israel Dublin award for Lifetime Achievement in the field of Suicide and a Career Achievement Award from the American Psychological Association. (Our Team n.d.). Reading about Marsha Linehan gave me hope. Marsha Linehan was diagnosed with Borderline Personality Disorder in her youth. She seemed to understand what was going on inside my head. She is quoted as stating:

The borderline individual is faced with an apparently irreconcilable dilemma. On the one hand, she has tremendous difficulties with self-regulation of affect and subsequent behavioral competence. She frequently but somewhat unpredictably needs a great deal of assistance, often feels helpless and hopeless, and is afraid of being left alone to fend for herself in a world where she has failed over and over again. Without the ability to predict and control her own well-being, she depends on her social environment to regulate her affect and behavior. On the other hand, she experiences intense shame at behaving dependently in a society that cannot tolerate dependency, and has learned to inhibit expressions of negative affect and helplessness whenever the affect is within controllable limits. (Linehan, 1993, p. 84)

Finally! Someone understood what I was feeling. I needed to find a therapist of this caliber. I was able to discover a local therapist who had studied under Linehan and was certified in Dialectical Behavior Therapy. I was forty years old and was only now getting the treatment I had needed my whole life. The therapist agreed to take me on as a new patient. I would have to pay out of pocket since my insurance would not cover the treatment. She took mercy on me and gave me a discounted rate since she was still building up clients in her new treatment location. She was one of two therapists near me specializing in DBT. In twenty years the amount of help for borderlines had only increased in my area by two therapists.

Ellen nicknamed my therapist T.L. She stated it stood for Therapy Lady. My therapist had a name that was easily confused with other people we knew. Going forward when Ellen and I would discuss our therapy sessions, T.L. was the name she would be known by. I bought my DBT skills training workbook and set off for my first meeting with my T.L.

None of my other therapists required book work or passed out worksheets. I enjoyed having to focus on homework and getting assignments on learning how to autoregulate myself. T.L shared her life story with me.

This was, in fact, her retirement job that she fell into out of her love of peoples' stories. She was the only therapist that was never shocked by my life. I never felt judged, which was a new feeling for therapy. It was refreshing to have a therapist treat you like a person. Most always treated me as if I belonged in a clock tower with a sniper rifle. My sessions would be broken into two parts. The first part would be talk therapy to deal with my past trauma. The second part would be book work teaching me skills to function in life. The brain is amazing in that new synapses can be formed and rerouted to learn new things. I was to be taught a new way to see things, and this would be the most difficult thing I have done my whole life.

I would look over my nightly homework trying to decipher the instructions. Darrin would read over my shoulder, and it would seem like such common sense to him. To me, it was if I was reading a foreign language. Is this what dyslexic kids felt like? I could eat fire, but I couldn't understand how to find my "wise mind." Wise mind is that part of your brain that combines logic and emotion to make thoughtful decisions (Linehan 2015).

T.L explained that I was about one incident away from completely splitting into Dissociative Identity Disorder. The trauma had shattered me into these multiple parts. I had these abused children of all different ages locked away inside that needed reassurance and love. Once these kids were healed, they would stop hijacking my emotions. My tantrums and fits of rage were childlike but with adult strength. Every time life would threaten me, one of these kids would emerge and lash out with the fury that they never could previously express.

I would walk out of jobs and quit without notice because the kids were running the show, not the adult. How did I find my wise mind adult voice? Was it the faint voice that was always in the back of my head? This would be found by healing the kids. I was to envision these parts in my mind and speak with them. However, I could not see them. My kids had built up this wall to hide behind and weren't coming out anytime soon. Why would they? They got their ice cream for breakfast and got to do whatever they wanted. The kids were happy living behind their wall. But the adult part of me was getting tired. I had been dealing with this struggle for forty years. During one session, T.L had a breakthrough. She got to meet one of the children inside. I came to a meeting after a bad fight with my boss at work. T.L stated that I was completely shut down. My mannerisms were different, along with my voice. There was no arguing with me. It was like arguing with a child. A child only sees their way. She had to find a way to get me to bring out the adult to discuss things further. I never felt any different, but she asked to record me so I could see the transformation myself. I wasn't ready for that and declined.

This breakthrough is when my therapist suggested I file for mental disability with Social Security. Was I disabled? I felt like I had been functioning. Then I realized I had been treading water for forty years, and nothing was getting better. I was still hustling check to check at various jobs similarly to how I hustled up drug money. Filing disability would give me access to the money I had personally paid into the social security system. I could still work while receiving Social Security. My Social Security check would just be offset by my wages. The monthly check would relieve the stress of constantly changing jobs and give me better insurance to pay for the full DBT treatment.

I went to the Social Security website, and it seemed pretty cut and dried. It stated that if you had one of these mental conditions, then you are eligible to receive your social security money early. I didn't just have one condition; I had five of them. I thought this should be an easy process. Nothing involving the government is an easy process. After filing, the Social Security office called me to offer me welfare instead of access to my Social Security funds. I didn't want other people to pay for me. I just wanted my own money that I had contributed. I thought that was the whole point of the system. At this time, I obtained a lawyer. Considering Social Security lawyers don't collect unless they win, I chose one on the highest floor of the most prominent downtown building.

The lawyer advised me that with no criminal record, suicide attempts, or records of being institutionalized that it would be a difficult case, but he would take it. The fact that I had never been caught, in either suicide attempts or my criminal activity, would be held against me. He also advised me to be on medication even though there were no medications for Borderline Personality Disorder. It was also suggested that I see a therapist that was a Ph.D. instead of a counselor.

It didn't matter to the Social Security Administration that my therapist was trained under the best and certified in DBT. Social Security stated that they needed proof I was indeed a borderline. They arranged for me to meet with one of their therapists. It was just the kind of therapist that I had chewed through in my twenties. All they cared about was the Ph.D. initials after his name. I called this therapist the War Doctor.

When I obtained his name, I started my research on him. He had been trained by the government in the art of interrogation. The American Board of Psychology had tried to remove his license twice for questionable actions but failed. The War Doctor was the man that was to cross-examine me to find flaws in my truth. The joke was on him. I had been trained to argue by the best. Training by the government was no match for the training I had learned from living with my mother. I was ready for our cage match. The whole meeting with the War Doctor was supposed to be at least forty-five minutes. I was out of his office in fifteen minutes. He notified Social Security that based on my combative nature and responses I was indeed a borderline along with other multiple diagnoses.

Next came a letter from Social Security stating that I no longer needed my retirement funds because they had located and Olive Garden 401K plan with $3,600. They suggested that I use these funds to retire on. I had to inform them that those funds were depleted last year when I purchased a used car. I didn't even address the absurdity of the amount being used for my retirement.

Finally, they agreed that I was indeed a person with Borderline Personality Disorder. This should have been the end, but sadly it was not. Now they decided to tell me how a borderline should live. Well, thank God. I had been trying to maintain for forty years, but apparently, Social Security was more knowledgeable about living with BPD. They suggested just obtaining a job with little interaction with people. At this point, I started to feel bad for the Social Security Administration. They were awful at their job.

I informed Social Security that I indeed had a job with little interaction with people. Then I presented them with my hospital bill for electrocuting myself at work because of my lack of focus. I am stuck in the middle. I cannot get along with others, which is my BPD. But when I work alone, my PTSD runs crazy, making me fearful and distracted. I am not a well-functioning employee. They agreed at this point to move my case to trial. The next trial date would be within three years.

Thinking about what my lawyer said, I made an appointment with my family doctor. Maybe things had changed in twenty years, and now there were medications. This only reinforced the rumors that I heard about judgment of Borderline Personality Disorder within the medical community. It was discussed that no one should advertise they have Borderline Personality Disorder because some medical personnel won't treat you. Leah was my counselor friend who had shared this knowledge with me.

Leah was a previous server coworker. She worked at Olive Garden while working on her social work degree. She was trained to be a counselor for domestic and sexual assault survivors. She shared with me that at a conference it was announced to the group of future counselors that they should avoid working with people who are borderlines. They state borderlines cause therapists to burn out since borderlines aren't easily fixable. So, because we are damaged and unable to make the therapists feel validated in their careers, we should be passed over for treatment? I was starting to understand why in twenty years, only two therapists in my area were skilled at working with Borderline Personality Disorder.

The look of shock on my family doctor's face when I informed her I was a borderline would be seared into my brain. She collapsed on her round wheeled chair and drifted backward away from me. She repeated over and over that there was no way I could be a borderline. Then she stated how this knowledge changed everything about how she treated me. This was a confusing statement. Until now, I only visited my family doctor once a year for a flu vaccine shot. How would my treatment change? I was still the same person.

I was trying to explain to her the process of me filing for disability. I would be mid-sentence, and she would interrupt me with invasive questions like, "Are you suicidal?! What are some thoughts that go through your head?". The look of fascination in her eyes I had seen in my prior therapists from my twenties. She was intrigued to have a real-life borderline in her office. I was once again behind glass like a zoo animal to be examined. Every visit after that would have Post-its on the computer monitor in all caps that read "BORDERLINE PERSONALITY DISORDER."

The doctor suggested I take antipsychotic medication that is prescribed for schizophrenia. There is an 80 percent chance of a drug-induced parkinsonism side effect. I would watch borderlines on YouTube complain about how they lost control of their tongue and had difficulty eating. Tardive dyskinesia is another side effect that produces these uncontrolled movements. Their muscles were so tight that they were in constant pain. Even if you stop the drug, the side effects stay. When I questioned my doctor about this, she laughed off the side effect. She also recommended electroconvulsive therapy. I didn't even know that shock treatment was still a thing we did as a society.

Voluntarily giving my brain a seizure, in the hopes of hitting it's reset button, was not an option that I found acceptable.

My T.L advised me once again that there were no drugs for borderlines. This was becoming apparently clear. However, Social Security did not understand this and stated that unless a person is medicated, they are not disabled because they have not honestly tried all solutions to fixing themselves. Statistics show that fewer than 1 percent of people fraudulently collect Social Security. (Social Security (n.d.). The approval rating for receiving Social Security is between 30 and 40 percent (Tritch 2015). That is a lot of people being denied the help they need. Maybe that's why the process takes a year. They hope the person asking for assistance dies within that time frame.

As a child, I was denied help. As an adult, I was now also getting denied assistance. Society has to stop letting people fall through the cracks. What if the teachers noticed the child that refused to go play outside on recess and questioned the kid? What if the neighbors investigated the yelling or the child fleeing a house? How about the relatives that never asked why the kids weren't allowed at family functions? Think about all the police that chased the same car every night or let me have a pass when I got pulled over intoxicated. What about the stigma that sends new therapists out in the world telling them not to interact with borderlines? Where is the help for the borderline? So many had a hand in creating the borderline, yet so few stepped up to offer life assistance.

The first year in DBT would fly by. I would find my voice and call out my mother for supporting those that sexually abused me. She would hang up the phone on me, and we would never speak again. I was the family outcast, and I was okay with that. I have reached a point where I do not want to be a part of that toxicity. It took the strength and love of Darrin for me to officially walk away, and I have been a stronger person because of it.

I still haven't finished my DBT workbook in this first year of DBT. T.L says that it's not a race and everyone learns at their own speed. I still see her every week and look forward to her empathy and warmth. A year in, and I'm starting to think that she meant it when she stated she wasn't going to give up on me. The important part is I'm trying to find a way to function, a way to breathe. My therapist gave me her cell phone number to call when I have my spin out moments of panic attacks or borderline rage. I thought at first, it was a sign of weakness to call her. I felt like I was bothering her. She states everyone feels like that in the beginning. I have learned that to call and ask for help is a sign of strength.

It takes courage to ask for help in this life. I asked for help as a child and was silenced. I gave up asking for help. Now I have to re-train myself to know that it is okay to need people. These are basic communication skills that I am learning at the age of forty-one. Darrin tells me he can see an improvement in my communication skills. He agreed for us to read communication books together to assist in strengthening our relationship. We still fight, but we are learning to do it healthily. He is learning my triggers, and I'm trying to learn the middle area of compromise that is needed in all human interaction. We were both damaged as children and are learning how to get along with each other in a healthy way. The upside to us both having damaged children inside us is we make great playmates for each other. He indulges in fun, childlike ideas like building a fort or decorating our living room with year-round Christmas lights.

The inner borderline is still racing and pushing me forward. The first draft of this book would be written in less than two months. I am getting ready to change jobs again. I grow tired of applying and starting new jobs, but I haven't fixed that part yet. I still want to constantly move but cannot tell if it's my flight/fight response or if I just hate where I live. I remain paralyzed, unable to make decisions. Some days I am still that person in the shower curtain aisle trying to figure out what my next step is.

The fractured parts are still hiding behind their walls, and with good reason. They endured a lot and learned that people were unreliable and couldn't be counted on for help. I still sit by that wall and talk to them. I can feel them on the other side of that wall.

Starting to feel anything is progress. I'm still waiting for the day they remove the first brick from that wall to look out. I want them to know that it's now safe. I want them to know that we all deserve love. I have hope. It took me forty-one years, but I finally have hope.

The thing I do know is that in this life, borderlines are not supposed to maintain relationships. Maybe the mental illness stigma is why borderlines don't have friends or the psychological help they need. I am grateful for all those that have impacted my life. My family was filled with the cruelest kind of people. Life is a balance, so it gave me wonderful friends and loved ones to offset the negative. I don't know if I will ever function well enough for a full-time job. I don't know if my marriage to Darrin will last forever. All I know is that in this life, people need to shine light in areas of darkness. Call people out for their bad behavior. Find peace and comfort in any which way possible. Above all else, protect the innocent. Love.

Others may disagree with my memories of these events, and that is their right. This is my story and not theirs. This is the story of a borderline. This is a story for The Neighbors.

References

Butler, L. (2016, January 01). Abuse and Neglect Increase a Child's Risk for Alcohol or Drug Addiction. Retrieved June 4, 2019, from https://twinlakesrecoverycenter.com/abuse-neglectincrease-childs-risk-alcohol-drug-addiction/

Crawford, C. (1979). Mommie Dearest. London: Granada.

Gardner, S. S. (2019, February 3). Breast Implant Safety: Risks and Safety Information About Silicone and Saline Breast Implants. Retrieved June 4, 2019, from https://www.webmd.com/beauty/breast-implant-safety

Linehan, M. M. (1993). Cognitive-behavioral treatment of borderline personality disorder (1st ed.). New York: Guilford Press.

Linehan, M. M. (2015). DBT skills training handouts and worksheets (2nd ed.). New York: The Guilford Press.

McBride, K. (2018, April 27). Narcissists Use "Gaslighting" to Control and Abuse. Retrieved June 5, 2019, from https://www.psychologytoday.com/us/blog/the-legacy-distortedlove/201804/narcissists-use-gaslighting-control-and-abuse

Our Team. (n.d.). Retrieved June 4, 2019, from https://depts.washington.edu/uwbrtc/ourteam/marsha-linehan/

Sack, D. (2015, December 21). The Destructive Power of Borderline Personality Disorder. Retrieved June 4, 2019, from https://www.psychologytoday.com/us/blog/where-science-meetsthe-steps/201512/the-destructive-power-borderline-personality-disorder

Severson, M. R.. (2012, October). Long-term health outcomes of childhood sexual abuse. Retrieved June 4, 2019, from https://www.americannursetoday.com/long-term-health-outcomes-of-childhood-sexual-abuse/

Social Security Administration (n.d.). Retrieved June 7, 2019, from https://www.ssa.gov/disabilityfacts/facts.html

Staff, F. E. (2018, November 13). Munchausen Syndrome by Proxy. Retrieved June 6, 2019, from https://familydoctor.org/condition/munchausen-syndrome-proxy/

Tritch, T. (2015, September 08). Busting the Myths About Disability Fraud. Retrieved June 7, 2019, from https://takingnote.blogs.nytimes.com/2015/09/08/busting-the-myths-about-disabilityfraud/

Van den Berg, J. (2018, June 18). Are Your Breast Implants Poisoning You? Retrieved June 4, 2019, from http://www.center4research.org/breast-implants-poisoning/

About the Author

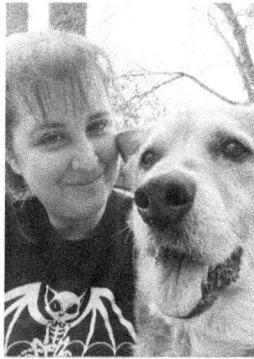

Cindy Collins has been living with Borderline Personality for over twenty years. She currently resides in Ohio with her husband, Darrin. They enjoy spending time with their dogs, Max and Bozworth. The spirits of dogs Maggie, Cherry, and Ginger are eternally loved and celebrated by the family. Cindy continuously works on her recovery through Dialectic Behavioral Therapy with her T.L. The marriage between Cindy and Darrin grows deeper in love with every passing day.